Scleroderma

Editor

MAUREEN D. MAYES

RHEUMATIC DISEASE CLINICS OF NORTH AMERICA

www.rheumatic.theclinics.com

Consulting Editor
MICHAEL H. WEISMAN

August 2015 • Volume 41 • Number 3

ELSEVIER

1600 John F. Kennedy Boulevard • Suite 1800 • Philadelphia, Pennsylvania, 19103-2899
http://www.theclinics.com

RHEUMATIC DISEASE CLINICS OF NORTH AMERICA Volume 41, Number 3

August 2015 ISSN 0889-857X, ISBN 13: 978-0-323-39354-6

Editor: Jennifer Flynn-Briggs
Developmental Editor: Casey Jackson

Rheumatic Disease Clinics of North America (ISSN 0889-857X) is published quarterly by Elsevier Inc., 360 Park Avenue South, New York, NY 10010-1710. Months of issue are February, May, August, and November. Business and editorial offices: 1600 John F. Kennedy Boulevard, Suite 1800, Philadelphia, PA 19103-2899. Periodicals postage paid at New York, NY and additional mailing offices. Subscription prices are USD 335.00 per year for US individuals, USD 579.00 per year for US institutions, USD 165.00 per year for US students and residents, USD 395.00 per year for Canadian individuals, USD 722.00 per year for Canadian institutions, USD 465.00 per year for international individuals, USD 722.00 per year for international institutions, and USD 230.00 per year for Canadian and foreign students/residents. To receive student/resident rate, orders must be accompanied by name of affiliated institution, date of term, and the *signature* of program/residency coordinator on institution letterhead. Orders will be billed at individual rate until proof of status received. Foreign air speed delivery is included in all *Clinics* subscription prices. All prices are subject to change without notice. **POSTMASTER:** Send address changes to *Rheumatic Disease Clinics of North America,* Elsevier Health Sciences Division, Subscription Customer Service, 3251 Riverport Lane, Maryland Heights, MO 63043. **Customer Service: 1-800-654-2452 (US and Canada). From outside of the US and Canada: 314-447-8871. Fax: 314-447-8029. For print support, e-mail: JournalsCustomerService-usa@elsevier.com**. **For online support, e-mail: JournalsOnline Support-usa@elsevier.com**.

Reprints. For copies of 100 or more of articles in this publication, please contact the Commercial Reprints Department, Elsevier Inc., 360 Park Avenue South, New York, New York, 10010-1710; Tel.: +1-212-633-3874, Fax: +1-212-633-3820, and E-mail: reprints@elsevier.com.

Rheumatic Disease Clinics of North America is covered in *MEDLINE/PubMed (Index Medicus), Current Contents/Clinical Medicine, Science Citation Index, ISI/BIOMED,* and *EMBASE/Excerpta Medica.*

Contributors

CONSULTING EDITOR

MICHAEL H. WEISMAN, MD
Cedars-Sinai Chair in Rheumatology, Director, Division of Rheumatology, Professor of Medicine, Cedars-Sinai Medical Center, Distinguished Professor, David Geffen School of Medicine at UCLA, Los Angeles, California

EDITOR

MAUREEN D. MAYES, MD, MPH
Professor of Internal Medicine, Elizabeth Bidgood Chair in Rheumatology, Division of Rheumatology and Clinical Immunogenetics, University of Texas-Houston Medical School, Houston, Texas

AUTHORS

MURRAY BARON, MD
Professor of Medicine, Division of Rheumatology, Jewish General Hospital, McGill University, Montreal, Quebec, Canada

LAURA CAPPELLI, MD
Division of Rheumatology, Johns Hopkins University School of Medicine, Baltimore, Maryland

LORINDA CHUNG, MD, MS
Department of Immunology and Rheumatology, Stanford University School of Medicine, Palo Alto, California

VANESSA C. DELISLE, MSc
Lady Davis Institute for Medical Research, Jewish General Hospital; Department of Educational and Counselling Psychology, McGill University, Montréal, Québec, Canada

CHRISTOPHER P. DENTON, PhD, FRCP
Centre for Rheumatology, UCL Royal Free Campus, London, United Kingdom

RINA S. FOX, MS, MPH
San Diego Joint Doctoral Program in Clinical Psychology, San Diego State University, University of California, San Diego, California

DANIEL E. FURST, MD
Emeritus Professor, Division of Rheumatology, Department of Medicine, David Geffen School of Medicine, University of California, Los Angeles, Los Angeles, California

SHADI GHOLIZADEH, MSc
San Diego Joint Doctoral Program in Clinical Psychology, San Diego State University, University of California, San Diego, California

LOÏC GUILLEVIN, MD
Department of Internal Medicine, Centre de Référence Maladies Systémiques et Auto-Immunes Rares, Hôpital Cochin, Assistance Publique-Hôpitaux de Paris, Université Paris Descartes, Paris, France

GENEVIEVE GYGER, MD
Assistant Professor, Division of Rheumatology, Jewish General Hospital, McGill University, Montreal, Quebec, Canada

LISA R. JEWETT, MSc
Lady Davis Institute for Medical Research, Jewish General Hospital; Department of Educational and Counselling Psychology, McGill University, Montréal, Québec, Canada

SINDHU R. JOHNSON, MD, PhD, FRCPC
Toronto Scleroderma Program, Division of Rheumatology, Department of Medicine, Toronto Western and Mount Sinai Hospitals; Institute of Health Policy, Management and Evaluation, University of Toronto, Toronto, Ontario, Canada

LINDA KWAKKENBOS, PhD
Lady Davis Institute for Medical Research, Jewish General Hospital; Department of Psychiatry, McGill University, Montréal, Québec, Canada

BROOKE LEVIS, MSc
Lady Davis Institute for Medical Research, Jewish General Hospital; Department of Epidemiology, Biostatistics, and Occupational Health, McGill University, Montréal, Québec, Canada

VANESSA L. MALCARNE, PhD
San Diego Joint Doctoral Program in Clinical Psychology, San Diego State University, University of California; Department of Psychology, San Diego State University, San Diego, California

MAUREEN D. MAYES, MD, MPH
Professor of Internal Medicine, Elizabeth Bidgood Chair in Rheumatology, Division of Rheumatology and Clinical Immunogenetics, University of Texas-Houston Medical School, Houston, Texas

KATHERINE MILETTE, MA
Lady Davis Institute for Medical Research, Jewish General Hospital; Department of Educational and Counselling Psychology, McGill University, Montréal, Québec, Canada

SARAH D. MILLS, MS
San Diego Joint Doctoral Program in Clinical Psychology, San Diego State University, University of California, San Diego, California

KATHLEEN B. MORRISROE, MBBS
Department of Rheumatology, St Vincent's Hospital, Fitzroy, Victoria, Australia

LUC MOUTHON, MD, PhD
Department of Internal Medicine, Centre de Référence Maladies Systémiques et Auto-Immunes Rares, Hôpital Cochin, Assistance Publique-Hôpitaux de Paris, Université Paris Descartes, Paris, France

SARANYA NANDAGOPAL, BA
Department of Dermatology, Stanford University School of Medicine, Redwood City, California

MANDANA NIKPOUR, MBBS, FRACP, FRCPA, PhD
Departments of Rheumatology and Medicine, St Vincent's Hospital, The University of Melbourne, Fitzroy, Victoria, Australia

JANET E. POPE, MD, MPH, FRCPC
Professor of Medicine, Department of Medicine, St. Joseph's Health Care, University of Western Ontario, London, Ontario, Canada

SUSANNA M. PROUDMAN, MBBS
Rheumatology Unit, Royal Adelaide Hospital; Discipline of Medicine, University of Adelaide, Adelaide, Australia

GLORIA SALAZAR, MD
Assistant Professor of Medicine, Division of Rheumatology and Clinical Immunogenetics, University of Texas Health Science Center at Houston, Houston, Texas

KATHERINE CULP SILVER, MD
Fellow, Adult and Pediatric Rheumatology, Medical University of South Carolina, Charleston, South Carolina

RICHARD M. SILVER, MD
Distinguished University Professor; Director, Division of Rheumatology and Immunology, Medical University of South Carolina, Charleston, South Carolina

VIRGINIA D. STEEN, MD
Division of Rheumatology, Allergy, and Immunology, Georgetown University School of Medicine, Washington, DC

EDWARD P. STERN, MBBS, MRCP
Centre for Rheumatology, UCL Royal Free Campus, London, United Kingdom

BRETT D. THOMBS, PhD
Lady Davis Institute for Medical Research, Jewish General Hospital; Departments of Psychiatry, Educational and Counselling Psychology, Epidemiology, Biostatistics, and Occupational Health, Medicine, Psychology, and School of Nursing, McGill University, Montréal, Québec, Canada

ANTONIA VALENZUELA, MD, MS
Department of Immunology and Rheumatology, Stanford University School of Medicine, Palo Alto, California

ELIZABETH R. VOLKMANN, MD, MS
Clinical Instructor, Division of Rheumatology, Department of Medicine, David Geffen School of Medicine, University of California, Los Angeles, Los Angeles, California

FREDRICK M. WIGLEY, MD
Division of Rheumatology, Johns Hopkins University School of Medicine, Baltimore, Maryland

Contents

Systemic sclerosis (SSc) is a complex autoimmune disease that occurs in a genetically susceptible host. Genetic studies performed so far reveal that multiple genetic loci contribute to disease susceptibility in SSc. The purpose of this review is to discuss the current knowledge of genetics in SSc by exploring the observational evidence, the different genetic studies, and their modalities as well as the most relevant genes discovered by these. The importance of gene expression variation and the different mechanisms that govern it, including the recently discovered field of epigenetics, are also explored, with an emphasis on microRNA.

Systemic sclerosis is a multisystem disorder with a high associated mortality. The hallmark abnormalities of the disease are in the immune system, vasculature, and connective tissue. Systemic sclerosis occurs in susceptible individuals and is stimulated by initiating events that are poorly understood at present. In order for the disease phenotype to appear there is dysfunction in the homoeostatic mechanisms of immune tolerance, endothelial physiology, and extracellular matrix turnover. The progression of disease is not sequential but requires simultaneous dysfunction in these normal regulatory mechanisms. Better understanding of the interplay of these factors is likely to contribute to improved treatment options.

The American College of Rheumatology (ACR)/European League Against Rheumatism (EULAR) criteria for the classification of systemic sclerosis (SSc) were developed to classify more patients with SSc for studies and improve on previous criteria. The new classification criteria have the following criteria: skin thickening of the fingers extending proximal to the metacarpophalangeal joints. Seven additive items are each given a numerical weight: skin thickening, fingertip lesions, telangiectasia, abnormal nail fold capillaries, lung involvement, Raynaud's phenomenon, and SSc-related autoantibodies. The ACR/EULAR classification criteria for SSc have good sensitivity and specificity but do not substitute for diagnostic criteria.

The skin is the most common organ system involved in patients with systemic sclerosis (SSc). Nearly all patients experience cutaneous symptoms, including sclerosis, Raynaud's phenomenon, digital ulcers, telangiectasias, and calcinosis. In addition to posing functional challenges, cutaneous symptoms are often a major cause of pain, psychological distress, and body image dissatisfaction. The present article reviews the main features of SSc-related cutaneous manifestations and highlights an evidence-based treatment approach for treating each manifestation. This article also describes novel treatment approaches and opportunities for further research in managing this important clinical dimension of SSc.

Raynaud phenomenon (RP) and associated digital ischemia can be among the most vexing clinical problems for patients with systemic sclerosis (scleroderma). Understanding the treatment approach to RP and associated ischemia and how to prevent digital ulcers is important for clinicians caring for these patients. This article reviews the management of RP and digital ischemic ulcers. The magnitude of the problem and pathophysiology of RP are first discussed, with an emphasis on recent advances in understanding of the disease process. Options for the practical pharmacologic and nonpharmacologic interventions for RP and digital ischemic ulcers are detailed.

Although scleroderma-associated interstitial lung disease (SSc-ILD) is a significant contributor to both morbidity and mortality, its pathogenesis is largely unclear. Pulmonary function tests and high-resolution computed tomographic scanning continue to be the most effective tools to screen for lung involvement and to monitor for disease progression. More research and better biomarkers are needed to identify patients most at risk for developing SSc-ILD as well as to recognize which of these patients will progress to more severe disease. Although immunosuppression remains the mainstay of treatment, antifibrotic agents may offer new avenues of treatment for patients with SSc-ILD in the future.

The gastrointestinal tract, affecting more than 90% of patients, is the internal organ most frequently involved in systemic sclerosis. Any part of the gastrointestinal tract can be affected, from the mouth to the anus. Patients often experience reduced quality of life and impaired social life. Although only 8% have severe gastrointestinal involvement, mortality is high in those patients. Recent studies on the pathophysiology of the disease highlight new mechanisms to explain gastrointestinal dysmotility, but treatment remains symptomatic. This article reviews the pathophysiology of the gastrointestinal tract and discusses the investigation and management of the disease.

Scleroderma renal crisis is a rare complication of systemic sclerosis (SSc) that remains severe. Prompt recognition and initiation of therapy with an angiotensin-converting-enzyme inhibitor offer the best chance to achieve a good outcome. SSc prevalence is poorly known, with disparities among countries.

Pulmonary arterial hypertension (PAH) is one of the leading causes of death in patients with systemic sclerosis (SSc). Given the high prevalence and poor survival of SSc-PAH, and that aggressive management of mild disease may be associated with better outcomes, screening is critical. Right heart catheterization (RHC) is the gold standard for the definitive diagnosis of PAH, and should be performed in those patients in whom this diagnosis is suspected. Once a diagnosis of PAH is confirmed by RHC, treatment with PAH-specific therapies should be initiated as soon as possible.

Systemic sclerosis (SSc; scleroderma) is a chronic autoimmune connective tissue disease characterized by microvascular obliteration and sclerosis of the skin and internal organs. Although the clinical hallmark of the disease is the appearance of taut tethering of the skin, one of the earliest manifestations of SSc is a painful symmetrical arthropathy ranging from minimal arthralgia to overt polyarthritis. Musculoskeletal (MSK) involvement in SSc occurs more frequently than expected. Arthralgia is the most commonly reported manifestation. Some of the existing composite and organ-specific indices of disease activity and/or disease severity in SSc include MSK manifestations.

Patients with systemic sclerosis (SSc; also called scleroderma) have to cope with not only the physical impacts of the disease but also the emotional and social consequences of living with the condition. Because there is no cure for SSc, improving quality of life is a primary focus of treatment and an important clinical challenge. This article summarizes significant problems faced by patients with SSc, including depression, anxiety, fatigue, sleep disruption, pain, pruritus, body image dissatisfaction, and sexual dysfunction, and describes options to help patients cope with the consequences of the disease.

RHEUMATIC DISEASE CLINICS OF NORTH AMERICA

RELATED INTEREST

Hand Clinics, February 2015 (Volume 31, Issue 1)
New Developments in Management of Vascular Pathology of the Upper Extremity
Steven L. Moran, Karim Bakri, and James P. Higgins, *Editors*

THE CLINICS ARE AVAILABLE ONLINE!
Access your subscription at:
www.theclinics.com

Foreword

Systemic Sclerosis

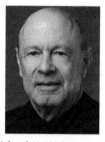

Michael H. Weisman, MD
Consulting Editor

Systemic Sclerosis (SSC), of all of the rheumatic diseases, is clearly the most challenging in terms of early diagnosis, understanding its pathogenesis, managing the different skin and internal organ phenotypes, and predicting prognosis. Today even the words renal crisis and scleroderma lung disease frighten the clinician because they know that patients die despite their best efforts to date. Nowhere is this truer than in the quest for its genetic associations where studies have been bedeviled by the lack of agreement regarding deep phenotype characterizations of study subjects. Stepping up to this challenge is Dr Maureen Mayes, who has assembled a strong group of experts in the field to bring the reader up-to-date on significant advances in this complex disease. These reviews focus on recognizing and identifying the clinical manifestations of disease, the mechanisms involved in SSC pathogenesis, the most recent findings regarding discovery of genetic susceptibility markers, and up-to-date management of the common and rare complications of this challenging disease. Maureen and her colleagues are certainly up to the task.

Michael H. Weisman, MD
Division of Rheumatology
Cedars-Sinai Medical Center
David Geffen School of Medicine at UCLA
8700 Beverly Boulevard
Los Angeles, CA 90048, USA

E-mail address:
Michael.Weisman@cshs.org

Rheum Dis Clin N Am 41 (2015) xiii
http://dx.doi.org/10.1016/j.rdc.2015.06.002
0889-857X/15/$ – see front matter © 2015 Published by Elsevier Inc.

rheumatic.theclinics.com

Preface

Systemic Sclerosis

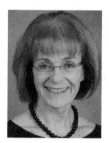

Maureen D. Mayes, MD, MPH
Editor

Since the last issue of *Rheumatic Disease Clinics of North America* on systemic sclerosis (SSc, scleroderma), there have been great advances in our understanding of the pathogenesis of this disease with the identification of multiple potentially promising targets for therapy. Remarkable progress has been made in determining genetic susceptibility factors and the different gene expression patterns that characterize disease tissue, which are summarized in the article entitled, "Genetics, Epigenetics, and Genomics of Systemic Sclerosis."

The article by Stern and Denton provides an elegant summary of current thought on SSc pathogenesis and the interplay of immune dysfunction, endothelial damage, and fibrotic pathways that contribute to disease. The article by Pope and Johnson presents the new 2013 classification system that more completely captures SSc patients, particularly those with early disease, for whom intervention may be more effective. Relevant case studies are provided to demonstrate how the new criteria can be applied to real world cases. The next seven articles discuss the major organ system manifestations with a focus on therapeutic options.

New in this issue, and of great importance to our patients, is a discussion of the psychosocial elements of SSc ("Psychosocial Aspects of Scleroderma"), and the burden these impose on our patients, including depression, anxiety, fatigue, sleep disruption, pain, pruritus, body image dissatisfaction, and sexual dysfunction.

These articles are meant to provide the interested clinician and researcher with the most current understanding of this complex and fascinating disease.

Contributors include scleroderma experts from the United States, Canada, the United Kingdom, Australia, and Europe reflecting the collaborative international effort for improved understanding and management of this disease. I am indebted to my

Rheum Dis Clin N Am 41 (2015) xv–xvi
http://dx.doi.org/10.1016/j.rdc.2015.06.001
0889-857X/15/$ – see front matter © 2015 Published by Elsevier Inc.

rheumatic.theclinics.com

colleagues for their dedication, expertise, and timely submissions. It is an honor to be part of this company.

Maureen D. Mayes, MD, MPH
Elizabeth Bidgood Chair in Rheumatology
Division of Rheumatology and Clinical Immunogenetics
University of Texas—Houston Medical School
6431 Fannin, Houston, TX 77030, USA

E-mail address:
Maureen.D.Mayes@uth.tmc.edu

Genetics, Epigenetics, and Genomics of Systemic Sclerosis

Gloria Salazar, MD, Maureen D. Mayes, MD, MPH*

KEYWORDS

- Genetics • Epigenetics • Systemic sclerosis • Scleroderma • Gene expression
- microRNA • miRNA • Splicing

KEY POINTS

- Multiple genes are associated with susceptibility to systemic sclerosis and can lead to alterations in innate and adaptive immunity, cell signaling, extracellular matrix, DNA or RNA degradation, and apoptosis or autophagy.
- There are several mechanisms (such as epigenetics and splicing mutations) that influence gene expression and are important for disease in addition to the genetic variants.
- Epigenetic mechanisms govern gene expression at different levels before translation. They are just being explored in systemic sclerosis and may help explain some of the missing heritability.

INTRODUCTION

Systemic sclerosis (SSc) is an autoimmune disease (AID) characterized by fibrosis of skin and internal organs as well as vasculopathy and immune dysregulation. SSc is a clinically heterogeneous disease and presents with 3 distinct subphenotypes: limited, diffuse, and "sine," based on the severity of skin involvement. This classification also reflects internal organ involvement, which can range from minimal to rapidly progressive disease resulting in premature death. Finally, SSc is characterized by the production of mutually exclusive antinuclear antibodies subtypes that are associated with different clinical manifestations, disease phenotypes, and prognosis.

SSc is a complex disease that entails abnormalities in several different pathways. Its pathogenesis is not well understood, but several studies have established that SSc occurs in a genetically susceptible host presumably after encountering environmental

Disclosures: The authors have no disclosures.
Division of Rheumatology and Clinical Immunogenetics, University of Texas Health Science Center at Houston, 6431 Fannin Street, MSB 5.270, Houston, TX 77030, USA
* Corresponding author.
E-mail address: Maureen.d.mayes@uth.tmc.edu

Rheum Dis Clin N Am 41 (2015) 345–366
http://dx.doi.org/10.1016/j.rdc.2015.04.001
0889-857X/15/$ – see front matter © 2015 Elsevier Inc. All rights reserved.

exposures or other external triggers.[1–3] Genetic studies performed so far reveal that multiple genetic loci contribute to disease susceptibility in SSc.[4] The purpose of this review is to discuss the current knowledge of SSc genetics by exploring the observational evidence, the different genetic studies performed to date, as well as the most relevant genes discovered by these. Also, the article explores the concept of gene expression variation and the recently discovered field of epigenetics.

INITIAL EVIDENCE OF THE GENETIC INFLUENCE IN SYSTEMIC SCLEROSIS

SSc is not inherited in a Mendelian fashion and, although its pathogenesis is unclear, it is thought that gene variants influence not only disease susceptibility but also differences in clinical expression and progression.[2] Here some of the initial observational evidence that supported the role of genetics in SSc is discussed.

Ethnic Associations

Differences in prevalence and clinical manifestations among different ethnic groups are evident and support the role of genetics in SSc. Some ethnic groups or subpopulations have higher prevalence of SSc compared with the general population. For example, the Choctaw tribe in Oklahoma is a population with a high prevalence of SSc (2 times higher than the expected prevalence) and displays a more homogeneous clinical and immunologic phenotype than is seen in the general population.[3,5]

Shared Genetic Background in Autoimmune Diseases

Several studies have noted that AIDs cluster in families (familial aggregation) and that there is co-occurrence in the same individual of 2 or more AIDs (individual aggregation or overlap syndromes) supporting the concept of a shared autoimmune genetic background among AIDs. In a cross-sectional study including 719 SSc patients, 38% had at least one other overlapping AID. The most frequent overlapping AIDs were autoimmune thyroid disease (AITD) (38%), rheumatoid arthritis (RA) (21%), and Sjogren syndrome (18%). Regarding the familial clustering of autoimmunity, 36% of the first-degree relatives had at least one AID, of which the most frequent were RA (18%) and AITD (9%),[6] suggesting that AIDs and their manifestations share genetic risk factors and support the role of genetic influences in SSc.

GENETIC STUDY MODALITIES

The most frequent type of DNA variation consists of a change in an individual nucleotide, known as a single-nucleotide polymorphism (SNP). These differences in the DNA sequence may or may not produce functional changes because of modification in the gene expression or alteration in the resulting protein.[7] In general, 2 basic approaches are used to study genetic associations: the candidate gene approach (CGA) and the genome-wide association study (GWAS). Both methodologies rely on the identification of SNPs and determine the likelihood that the variant occurs more or less frequently in the cases than in the controls (communicated in the form of an odds ratio).[8]

To date, genetic studies have identified SSc susceptibility factors involved in the immune system as well as genes in pathways that play a role in vascular damage and fibrotic processes.[1,3]

Candidate Gene Approach

CGA studies aim to determine specific SNPs associated with disease. Candidate genes are chosen either because they have been associated with other AIDs or because they make biological sense (ie, are part of pathways hypothesized to be important for the disease pathogenesis). Therefore, the major advantage of the CGA is that one can test for a particular SNP with known functional consequences.[8–10] Using this strategy, several novel genetic risk factors for SSc or its clinical phenotypes have been identified, and these polymorphisms tend to cluster in specific pathways. However, CGA studies are often limited by small cohorts and lack of replication. Genes discovered by CGA are reviewed in **Tables 1–3**.

Genome-Wide Association Studies, Meta–Genome-Wide Association Studies, and Pan-Meta–Genome-Wide Association Studies

GWAS, as opposed to CGA, perform genetic profiling of patients compared with controls by screening SNPs across the entire genome without making a priori assumptions about what loci are likely to be involved in the disease. Therefore, a major advantage to the GWAS approach is that it is unbiased and can identify novel genes that were not previously suspected to be disease-associated, leading to the identification of new pathogenetic mechanisms and yielding many new genetic susceptibility loci.[8,11] However, a GWAS is limited by the used platform because most provide approximately 80% coverage for common polymorphisms in the human genome and miss unusual variants. Another limitation is that GWAS usually investigate SNPs that are in strong linkage disequilibrium with other SNPs and serve as proxies for them so that the identified SNPs are just a tag for the yet to be identified causal allele.[12]

To date, several GWAS in SSc have confirmed that the major histocompatibility complex (MHC) is the strongest susceptibility loci for SSc. Also, multiple non-MHC susceptibility loci have been identified and the most robust associations are in genes related to innate immunity as well as B-cell and T-cell activation, which confirmed the concept that SSc is an AID. In 2010, the first robust GWAS in SSc was published that included 2296 SSc patients and 5171 healthy controls from the Netherlands, Germany, Spain, and the United States. It revealed that the strongest association was observed at the 6p21 locus corresponding to the MHC. The SNP rs6457617, located in HLA*DQB1, showed the strongest association. In addition, 5 non-human leukocyte antigen (HLA) loci reached genome-wide significance: TNPO3/IRF5, STAT4, CD247, CDH7, and EXOC2/IRF4 (see **Table 1; Table 4**).[13] Subsequent GWAS with a high-resolution marker revealed associations at PSORS1C1 (HLA region), TNIP1, and ras homolog gene family, member B (RHOB) (see **Tables 2 and 3**).[14]

To increase the statistical power to identify low-frequency variants as well as to perform subphenotype analysis, it has become popular to merge data from 2 or more published GWAS and perform a meta-analysis, also known as meta-GWAS (MGWAS).[15]

As mentioned before, observational studies support the theory that AIDs share a genetic background. Following this hypothesis, some investigators have merged and analyzed GWAS performed in different AIDs, a concept known as pan-meta-GWAS (PMGWAS).[15] For example, a PMGWAS, including systemic lupus erythematosus (SLE) and SSc cohorts, increased the sample size to a total of 21,109 (6835 cases) and found, apart from the already known shared susceptibility loci for both diseases, 3 more that were new to SSc (KIAA0319L, PXK, and JAZF1, see **Table 4**).[16]

Altogether, these approaches have identified genetic variants T-cell signaling and interferon (IFN) signaling pathways as associated with SSc susceptibility and revealed roles in apoptosis, DNA, or RNA degradation and autophagy pathways.[10]

Table 1
Adaptive, innate immunity and interferon pathway genes associated with systemic sclerosis

Gene	Product	Location	Polymorphisms	Approach	Phenotype	Function	References
Innate immunity and IFN pathways							
IRF5	Interferon regulatory factor 5	7q32	rs3757385 rs2004640 rs10954213 rs4728142 rs2280714 rs10488631 rs12537284	GWAS CGA	GSSc dcSSc ATA ILD	Regulates expression of IFN-dependent genes	13,48–52
IRF7	Interferon regulatory factor 7	11p15	rs4963128 rs702966 rs1131665	CGA	ACA	Same	53
IRF8	Interferon regulatory factor 8	16q24	rs11642873 rs11117425 rs11644034 rs12711490	GWAS	lcSSc ACA	Modulates TLR signaling, regulates IFN gene expression	21
NLRP1	NACHT, LRR, and PYD domains-containing protein 1	17p13	rs8182352	CGA	ATA ILD	Interacts with caspases 2 and 9, crucial for the inflammatory response	54
Adaptive immunity							
BANK1	Scaffold protein with ankyrin repeat	4q24	rs3733197 rs10516487 rs17266594 rs3733197	CGA	GSSc dcSSc ATA	B-cell-specific scaffold protein, involved in B-cell activation	42,55

Gene	Gene name	Locus	SNP	Method	Disease	Function	References
BLK	B-lymphocyte kinase	8p23	rs13277113, rs2736340, rs13277113	CGA, MA	GSSc, ACA, lcSSc	Downstream BCR signaling	56–58
IRAK1	Interleukin-1 receptor associated kinase-1	Xq28	rs1059702	CGA	GSSc, ILD, dcSSc, ATA	Regulates NF-kB through TCR	24,59
STAT4	Signal transducer and activator of transcription 4	2q32	rs7574865, rs3821236, rs10168266, rs11889341, rs8179673, rs10181656, rs6752770	CGA, GWAS	GSSc, lcSSc	Transduces IL-12, IL-23. Promotes Th1 cells and negatively regulates Th2	13,14,41,60–62
CD247	T-cell receptor ζ (CD3ζ) subunit	1q22	rs2056626	CGA, GWAS	GSSc, dcSSc, lcSSc	Key component of TCR signaling function	13,14,63
TBX21	T-box 21 protein (T-bet)	17q21	rs11650354	CGA	GSSc	Critical transcription factor for Th1 development	60
FOXP3	Forkhead box P3	Xp11	rs3761548, rs2280883	CGA	GSSc, lcSSc, ACA	Master regulator of Treg cells	25

Abbreviations: BCR, B-cell receptor; GSSc, global systemic sclerosis; IL-12, interleukin 12; IL-23, interleukin 23; ILD, interstitial lung disease; lcSSc, limited cutaneous systemic sclerosis; NF-kB, nuclear factor κ light-chain enhancer of activated B cells; TCR, T-cell receptor; Th1, T-helper 1; Th2, T-helper 2; TLR, Toll-like receptor; Treg, T-regulatory cells.

Table 2
Signaling pathways and cytokine genes associated with systemic sclerosis

Gene	Product	Location	Polymorphisms	Approach	Phenotype	Function	References
Signaling pathways							
TNFAIP3	Tumor necrosis factor α-induced protein 3	6q23	rs5029939 rs2230926	CGA GWAS	GSSc dcSSc ATA ILD PAH	Negative feedback regulation of the NF-kB pathway	64–66
TNIP1	TNFAIP3-interacting protein 1	5q33	rs2233287 rs4958881 rs3792783	GWAS	GSSc	Same	14
PTPN22	Protein tyrosine phosphatase nonreceptor type 22	1p13	rs2476601	CGA	GSSc ATA	Regulates TCR signal transduction	67–69
TNFSF4	Tumor necrosis factor (ligand) superfamily, member 4 (OX40L)	1q25	rs1234314 rs2205960 rs844648 rs4916334 rs10798269 rs12039904 rs8448644 rs844665	CGA	GSSc lcSSc ACA ATA ARA	Binds to OX-40 on T cells (costimulatory signal) vital for T-cell activation	70–72
CD226	Cluster of differentiation 226 (DNAX accessory molecule 1)	18q22	rs763361	CGA	GSSc dcSSc ATA ILD	T-cell costimulatory pathways	73,74
SOX5	SRY (sex determining region Y)-box 5	12p12	rs11047102	MGWAS	ACA	Regulation of embryonic development, determination of cell fate, and chondrogenesis	21

Gene	Gene name	Location	SNP	Study	Subset	Function	Ref
NOTCH4	NOTCH 4	6p21	rs443198 rs9296015	CGA MGWAS	ACA ATA	Controls cell fate decisions	21
GRB10	Growth factor receptor-bound protein 10	7p12	rs12540874	CGA MGWAS	lcSSc	Adaptor protein involved in multiple signaling pathways	21
Cytokines and chemokines							
IL1B	Interleukin 1β	2q14	rs1143627 rs16944	CGA	GSSc	Crucial for inflammatory responses	75
IL2RA	Interleukin-2 receptor subunit α	10p15	rs2104286	CGA	ACA	Treg marker	76
IL6	Interleukin 6	7p21	rs2069840	MA	lcSSc	Crucial role in both adaptive and innate immunity	77
IL10	Interleukin 10	1q32	N/A	CGA	GSSc	Anti-inflammatory cytokine	78,79
IL12RB2	Interleukin-12 receptor subunit β-2	1p31	rs3790567	GWAS	GSSc	Promotes Th differentiation into Th1 cells	80
IL13	Interleukin 13	5q31	rs2243204	CGA	GSSc	Secreted by activated Th2 cells shown to be involved in fibrosis	81
IL21	Interleukin 21	4q27	rs6822844 rs907715	CGA	GSSc	Potent immunomodulatory cytokine	82
IL23R	Interleukin 23 receptor	1p31	rs11209026 rs11465804	CGA	ATA	Stabilize the Th17 phenotype	83
MCP1 (CCL2)	Monocyte chemotactic protein 1 (CCL2)	17q12	N/A	CGA	GSSc	Recruits monocytes, memory T cells, and dendritic cells to sites of inflammation	84

Abbreviations: ARA, anti-RNA polymerase III; GSSc, global systemic sclerosis; ILD, interstitial lung disease; lcSSc, limited cutaneous systemic sclerosis; MA, meta-analysis; NF-κB, nuclear factor κ light-chain enhancer of activated B cells; PAH, pulmonary arterial hypertension; TCR, T-cell receptor; Th1, T-helper 1; T-helper 2; Th17, T-helper 17; Treg, T-regulatory cells.

Table 3
Extracellular matrix and other genes associated with systemic sclerosis

Gene	Product	Location	Polymorphisms	Approach	Phenotype	Function	References
Extracellular matrix							
FBN1	Fibrillin 1	15q21	N/A	CGA	GSSc	Glycoprotein, structural component of microfibrils	85,86
CSK	C-Src tyrosine kinase	15q24	rs1378942	GWAS	GSSc	Inactivates the c-Src kinases that lead to fibrosis	65
CTGF (CCN2)	Connective tissue growth factor	6q23	rs6918698	CGA	GSSc	Promotes fibroblast proliferation and ECM production	87
SPARC (osteonectin)	Secreted protein acidic and rich in cysteine	5q33	N/A	CGA GWAS	GSSc	Modulates cell-matrix interactions	88
Other genes							
DNASE1L3	Deoxyribonuclease 1-like 3	3p14	rs35677470	IC	ACA	DNA fragmentation during apoptosis	1
ATG5	Autophagy protein 5	6q21	rs9373839	IC	GSSc	Protein necessary for autophagy	1
RHOB	Ras homolog family, protein B	2p24	rs13021401 rs342070	GWAS	GSSc	Cell migration	14
PXK	PX serine threonine kinase	3P14	rs2176082	PMGWAS	ACA	Trafficking of the EGFR	16
JAZF1	Juxtaposed with another zinc finger protein 1	7p15	rs1635852	PMGWAS	GSSc	Associated with skeletal frame size and height, likely related to bone morphogenesis and collagen deposition	16
KIAA0319L	KIAA0319-like protein	1p34	rs2275247	PMGWAS	lcSSc	Unknown	16
MECP2	Methyl-CpG binding Protein 2	Xq28	rs17435	CGA	GSSc dcSSc	Binds to methylated DNA, transcriptional regulation of methylated genes	24
PSORS1C1	Psoriasis susceptibility 1 candidate 1	6p21	rs3130573	GWAS	GSSc	Unknown	14

Abbreviations: EGFR, epidermal growth factor receptor; GSSc, global systemic sclerosis; lcSSc, limited cutaneous systemic sclerosis; NF-kB, nuclear factor κ light-chain enhancer of activated B cells.

Table 4
Intergenic regions associated with systemic sclerosis

Gene	Product	Location	Polymorphisms	Approach	Phenotype	Function	References
SCHIP-IL12A	N/A	3q25	rs77583790	IC	GSSc lcSSc ACA	Unknown	[1]
TREH-DDX6	N/A	11q23	rs7130875	IC	GSSc	Unknown	[1]
TNPO3-IRF5	N/A	7q32	rs12537284	GWAS	GSSc	Unknown	[13]
CDH7	N/A	18q22	rs10515998	GWAS	GSSc	Unknown	[13]
EXOC2-IRF4	N/A	6p25	rs4959270	GWAS	GSSc	Unknown	[13]

Abbreviations: GSSc, global systemic sclerosis; lcSSc, limited cutaneous systemic sclerosis.

Immunochip

The Immunochip (IC) is a custom SNP genotyping array that provides high-density mapping of AID-associated loci for large cohorts at reduced costs and that specifically targets rare as well as common variants. It can be considered a hybrid between the CGA and GWAS approaches designed specifically for AIDs because only SNPs that are known to be involved in AIDs are examined. The IC array platform contains 196,524 variants across 186 known autoimmunity risk loci.[12] In 2014, the first SSc IC study was published, following in the footsteps of other AIDs. It validated the importance of the HLA region and found new associations, including DNASE1L3, the SCHIP1-IL12A locus, and ATG5, as well as a suggestive association between the TREH-DDX6 locus and SSc (see **Tables 3** and **4**).[1]

KNOWN GENETIC ASSOCIATIONS WITH SYSTEMIC SCLEROSIS
Major Histocompatibility Complex Region—Human Leukocyte Antigen Genes

The strongest genetic association observed in SSc is within the MHC region. The MHC complex located on chromosome 6p21.31 is characterized by the extraordinarily polymorphic HLA alleles and other immunoregulatory genes. Allelic variation in this region has been associated with a wide range of AIDs, including SLE, RA, ankylosing spondylitis, and others.

Polymorphisms in the HLA region have been extensively linked to SSc susceptibility, and there are multiple studies that confirm that some HLA types are associated with a general susceptibility to SSc, whereas others are more strongly related to particular disease subtypes.[2] Similarly, some of these associations are common to several ethnicities, whereas others are unique to a specific population group.[17–19]

As previously mentioned, the *HLA-DQB1* gene region conferred the strongest susceptibility for SSc per GWAS. A large multiethnic GWAS published in 2009 revealed that different HLA genotypes not only influence disease susceptibility but also are associated with autoantibody expression and vary according to ethnicity. The strongest positive class II associations with SSc in whites and Hispanics were the *DRB1*1104, DQA1*0501,* and *DQB1*0301* alleles. In blacks, SSc associated with *DRB1*0804, DQA1*0501,* and *DQB1*0301*. *DPB1*1301* showed the highest odds ratio for antitopoisomerase (ATA) (odds ratio = 14) and anticentromere (ACA) was associated with *DQB1*0501* and *DQB1*26*.[20]

Major Histocompatibility Complex Region Non-human Leukocyte Antigen Genes

NOTCH 4 and PSORS1C1 are 2 genes associated with SSc that are also located in the MHC region but do not code for HLA proteins (see **Table 2**). For example, NOTCH4 encodes a transmembrane protein that plays a role in developmental processes by controlling cell fate decisions and has been implicated in pathways that induce pulmonary fibrosis via transforming growth factor β (TGF-β). The Notch signaling pathway also controls key functions in vascular smooth muscle and endothelial cells.[21] NOTCH4 polymorphisms have been associated with ACA- and ATA-positive patients.[21] Little is known about PSORS1C1 other than it is also associated with psoriasis.[22]

Non-major Histocompatibility Complex Genes

Multiple non-MHC loci have been associated with SSc. Here the most notable genes discovered to date according to their role in metabolic pathways are reviewed.

Innate immunity and interferon pathway genes

A growing body of evidence has provided a new paradigm for understanding autoimmunity. Type I IFN is now thought to be a central mediator of innate immunity and therefore key for multiple AIDs, SSc included. IFN microarray studies first discovered a key role of the type I IFN in the pathogenesis of SLE and SS through observation of an IFN "signature" in peripheral blood cells (PBC) and salivary glands. Recent data investigating immunologic alterations occurring in early SSc by transcriptional profiling of PBC demonstrated a similar "IFN signature."[23] Type I and II IFN are well-known immunomodulators that can also regulate collagen production and therefore are thought to play a key role in the pathogenesis of SSc.[21] **Table 1** lists the most notable innate immune genes involved in SSc.

Adaptive immunity

Associations between defects in B-cell and T-cell signaling components and SSc pathogenesis have also been described. T-cell- and B-cell-related gene polymorphisms highlight the importance of these cells and the adaptive immune system in SSc susceptibility. **Table 1** lists the adaptive immunity genes and their reported associations with SSc.

Cell signaling pathways, cytokines, and chemokines

Variants in genes that code for several cytokines and cytokine receptors as well as various other signaling pathways have been reported to be associated with SSc. They underscore the importance of the immune system and other nonimmune signaling pathways, such as cell fate decisions in the pathophysiology of SSc. These genes are summarized in **Table 2**.

Extracellular matrix genes and others

Several genes involved in extracellular matrix (ECM) deposition have been implicated in the pathogenesis of SSc. Genetic studies in SSc have also revealed the importance of genes and pathways that were previously not considered, such as DNASE1L3 (involved in DNA fragmentation) and ATG5 (involved in autophagy), which implicate 2 novel pathways not previously considered to be important in SSc pathogenesis.[1] Three other novel genes with various functions involved in SSc were discovered by the PWGWAS (see **Table 3**).[16]

The X chromosome

To date, there are 3 genes associated with SSc susceptibility that are located on the X chromosome: IRAK1, FOXP3, and MECP2.[24,25] Considering the strong female predilection of SSc, these genes could be of great importance to its pathophysiology. IRAK1 and FOXP3 are vital for T-cell function (see **Table 1**). Interestingly, MECP2 has a key role in DNA methylation and therefore is part of the epigenetic mechanisms for gene regulation (see **Table 3**).[24]

OTHER SOURCES OF GENETIC VARIATION

Very few of the SSc-associated SNPs are found in coding (exonic) regions, but instead are in intronic areas or intragenic regions. It is now clear that there is a complex network of molecular interactions orchestrating gene expression and that these differences are strongly heritable. Genetic mutations that alter any step in this genomic regulatory network can affect gene expression and contribute to regulatory variation. Abnormal gene expression is increasingly recognized as a cause for many disease processes.[26,27]

Intronic and Intergenic Mutations

For many years it was thought that the DNA regions that do not code for proteins (known as "noncoding" regions) were not functionally relevant and terms such as "gene deserts" or "junk DNA" were coined for them; however, several studies throughout the years have challenged this idea. GWAS in various diseases (SSc included) have discovered several disease susceptibility loci in these regions and, in fact, the vast majority of variants discovered to date are found in noncoding regions (88%).[27–29] It has therefore become increasingly clear that these regions are actually of great importance because they are an integral part of a complicated network that regulates gene expression.

These noncoding regions include 2 types of DNA sequences: introns and intergenic regions. Introns are nucleotide sequences within a gene that are removed by RNA splicing and eliminated before the final gene product or mature RNA is generated. Intergenic regions are stretches of DNA located between genes. Mutations in both have been discovered in SSc and various other diseases. Mutations in introns can cause a premature stop codon, which can generate a truncated (shortened) or abnormally long nonfunctional or poorly functional protein. Mutations in intergenic regions are thought to affect the normal function of silencer or enhancer sequences. Altering a gene promoter will lead to abnormal gene expression that in turn can cause a disease state.

Multiple polymorphisms of introns located in protein coding genes have been described in SSc and most GWAS hits are actually intronic. Mutations in several intergenic regions have also been described. One example includes the region between SCHIP1 and IL12A that has been strongly associated with SSc, particularly with the limited type, and was also identified in celiac disease by IC.[1] Another suggestive association was identified in the 11q23 intergenic region between TREH and DDX6. DDX6 is an RNA helicase that is important for efficient miRNA-induced gene silencing and has been shown to regulate vascular endothelial growth factor under hypoxic conditions, which might provide a clue to the vasculopathy and fibrosis characteristic of this disease, as well as support the importance of epigenetics in SSc.[1] **Table 4** lists well-known intergenic regions described as susceptibility variants in SSc.

Splicing Mutations

Recognizing which genomic regions are intronic and which are exonic is key for proper gene expression and this depends on a process called "splicing." Splicing entails the modification of the pre-mRNA transcript by removing introns and joining the exons. The splicing process occurs through a ribonucleoprotein complex known as the spliceosome. This complex is formed by highly dynamic associations and dissociations of hundreds of particles. Many elements can affect the splicing process, and understanding how the spliceosome can successfully distinguish exons from introns is vital to decoding gene expression.[30,31] Splicing mutations can occur, and when this happens, they can induce exon skipping, form new exon/intron boundaries, or activate new cryptic exons. Mutations in introns can also lead to splice mutations. It is estimated that the very high number of currently unclassified genetic alterations may be due to unrecognized gene splicing abnormalities.[30,31] In SSc, research is barely scratching the surface of these intricate mechanisms and their implication for the disease. One study found that an enzyme named Lysyl hydroxylase 2 (LH2), which is vital to the alternatively splicing in collagen biosynthesis, might play an important role in SSc. Changes in the pattern of LH2 alternative splicing can favor increased inclusion of an exon that should be excised, thereby increasing the levels of a long transcript that is linked to SSc.[32]

Expression Quantitative Trait Locus

Given that gene expression levels are considered a heritable and quantitative trait, it is natural to infer that there are associations between gene expression and genotype that can be statistically established and would help identify loci that are associated or linked to gene expression levels. This concept would be especially useful for associations observed in noncoding regions that previously did not have a functional explanation. It was this idea that generated a technique called expression quantitative trait locus (eQTL) mapping, which is used to determine the effects of genetic variants on gene expression levels.[26] eQTL studies have established convincing relationships between genetic variants and gene expression by contrasting mean differences in phenotypes among genotypes.[33] The eQTL analyses have been successful in mapping variants to gene expression in several cell types, providing a better understanding of the genetics of gene expression and revealing functional impacts of variants associated with complex traits and diseases.[28]

Gene variants in regulatory regions were classified by eQTL into 2 types based on the relationship between the genomic location of the mutation and the gene or genes they regulate. A cis-regulatory variant alters expression of an associated or nearby gene (local effects). These variants lie either in the basal promoter region located near the transcription start site or in an enhancer located in noncoding sequences surrounding the transcribed region. On the other hand, a trans-regulatory change regulates expression of genes that are not contiguous and many times are even on different chromosomes (distant effects). eQTL studies show that 25% to 35% of variants are consistent with cis-regulatory effects, and the remaining are classified as trans-acting. Interestingly, there is a striking similarity in the amount of cis- and trans-regulatory variation found in genomes from diverse organisms, which suggests common gene regulatory mechanisms that were preserved through evolution.[27] To date, eQTL studies have not been performed in SSc but have been successful for other AIDs, such as SLE, making it an attractive future direction in SSc genetics research.[34]

Epigenetics

Considering that genetics alone is unable to fully account for SSc risk and the polymorphisms that were discovered in noncoding regions, SSc research over the past 5 years has evolved to explore a new field known as epigenetics.[3,10] Epigenetic variants are defined as the changes in gene function that are inheritable but do not entail a DNA sequence change. Apart from the baseline genomic milieu and the interplay between silencer and enhancer sequences, the epigenetic mechanisms help explain genetic variation given their vital role in gene expression regulation and can account for part of the missed heritability.[10] Some of the epigenetic mechanisms known to date include DNA methylation, histone modification, microRNA (miRNA), and long noncoding RNAs (lncRNA) variants. Disruption of any step in this complicated chain of regulatory events can lead to pathologic abnormality. Current knowledge in this field is briefly discussed.

MicroRNA and long noncoding RNA

MiRNAs are small, 19 to 23-nucleotide-long, noncoding RNAs that are part of a complicated network that regulates the expression of protein-coding genes. MiRNAs are predicted to regulate up to one-third of all human protein-coding genes, and most do so by negatively blocking their target mRNA after transcription, therefore leading to degradation or repression of translation.[35] MiRNA regulate multiple key pathways that when dysregulated can lead to inflammation, fibrosis, and angiogenesis. Various miRNA have been described to be either upregulated or downregulated in tissues of SSc patients compared with healthy controls, including whole skin, fibroblasts, or serum. **Table 5** depicts the known differentially expressed miRNA in SSc to date. Interestingly, some of these miRNA are also dysregulated in other fibrotic diseases, such as renal fibrosis or liver cirrhosis. For example, 2 miRNAs that are shared by multiple fibrotic diseases include the miR-21 and miR-29 families.[36–38]

Only miRNA that have been recapitulated by a second method other than microarray are listed in **Table 5**. Using biocomputational prediction algorithms, which are well-established screening tools for miRNA profiling, the miRNAs discovered to date in SSc are usually predicted to target fibrotic pathways such as TGF-β.[39] Target validation is an important step in miRNA research; it involves proving in vitro that a miRNA truly blocks the mRNA that it was predicted to target in silico. **Table 5** lists the targets that have been validated as opposed to just predicted.

LncRNAs, as the name depicts, are longer RNAs, usually greater than 200 nucleotides. LncRNA are also a recently recognized genetic expression regulation mechanism. This field is in its infancy, but so far it appears very promising because several lncRNA are reported to regulate immune responses.[40] This mechanism, therefore, needs to be further investigated in SSc.

Other epigenetic mechanisms

DNA methylation occurs when a methyl group is added to cytosine phosphate guanine (CpG) dinucleotides that are concentrated in regions called "CpG islands," usually located within promoter regions. This addition promotes a condensed DNA configuration, blocking accessibility to transcriptional activators and thereby inhibiting gene transcription. Histone modification occurs when histones are acetylated, phosphorylated, or methylated, influencing the accessibility of chromatin to transcription factors. These mechanisms have been explored to some degree in SSc and are vital for gene regulation expression. Advances in methylation and histone modification in SSc were recently reviewed in great detail by Broen and colleagues.[10]

Gene-Gene Interactions

The contribution of individual genes to the genetic risk for SSc is modest. Multiple loci are involved and probably interact, increasing the risk. It was not until recently that genetic research in SSc started to combine genetic data to determine whether some variants could have an additive risk for SSc susceptibility when found in the same individual. An additional finding that justifies this hypothesis is that many SSc candidate genes map to the same biological pathways. The first successful attempt to study gene-gene interaction in SSc showed that STAT4 (rs7574865) and IRF5 (rs2004640) variants form an additive risk for development of SSc and interstitial lung disease.[41] This analysis was then repeated, including the BANK1 polymorphisms, and was

Table 5
Dysregulated microRNA in systemic sclerosis

miRNA	Location	Predicted Targets	Validated	Induced or Suppressed by	Tissue	Method	Phenotype	References
Downregulated								
let-7a	9q22	COL1A1 COL1A2	Yes	Unknown	Skin Serum Fibroblasts	TPCR PCRa	GSSc	89
miR-29a	7q32	COL1A1 COL1A2 COL3A1	Yes	TGF-β PDGF-B IL-4	Skin Serum Hair	TPCR	GSSc	90–92
miR-30b	8q24	PDGFR-β	Yes	TGF-β	Serum	TPCR	GSSc dcSSc	93
miR-125b	11q24	SMAD5 CD28	No	Unknown	Skin	mirA TPCR	GSSc	90,94
miR-129-5p	7q32	COL1A1	Yes	Unknown	Fibroblasts	PCRa TPCR	GSSc	95
miR-145	5q32	SMAD3	No	Unknown	Skin Fibroblasts	TPCR mirA	GSSc	90,94
miR-150	19q13	Integrin β3	Yes	Unknown	Skin Serum Fibroblasts	TPCR PCRa ISH	GSSc	96
miR-196a	17q21	COL1A1 COL1A2	No	TGF-β	Hair Skin Serum Fibroblasts	TPCR PCRa ISH	GSSc dcSSc P&U	97–99

miRNA	Location	Target genes						Ref
miR-206	6p12	TGFB1 TGFB2 SMAD5 Integrin α2	No	Unknown	Skin	mirA TPCR	GSSc	90,94
Upregulated								
let-7g	3p21	COL1A2 COL2A1 COL5A2 TGFB2R	No	Unknown	Skin	mirA TPCR	GSSc	94
miR-7	9q21	COL1A2	No	TSP-2	Skin Fibroblasts	PCRa ISH	GSSc	100
miR-21	17q23	SMAD7	Yes	TGF-β	Skin Fibroblasts	TPCR mirA	GSSc	90,101
miR-92a	13q31	MMP1	No	TGF-β	Serum Fibroblasts	TPCR	GSSc < TA	102
miR-142-3p	17q22	Integrin αV	No	TGF-β	Serum	TPCR	GSSc	103

Abbreviations: COL1A1, collagen 1 α1; COL1A2, collagen 1 α2; COL3A1, collagen 3 α1; GSSc, global systemic sclerosis; IL-4, interleukin 4; ISH, in situ hybridization; mirA, miRNA array; MMP1, matrix metalloproteinase 1; P&U, pits and ulcers; PCRa, PCR array; PDGF-B, platelet derived growth factor β; PDGFR-β, platelet-derived growth factor receptor β; TA, telangiectasias; TGFB1, TGF β1; TGFB2R, transforming growth factor β receptor II; TPCR, targeted polymerase chain reaction; TSP-2, thrombospondin 2.

able to display an additive effect for diffuse SSc susceptibility. In a subsequent analysis, an NLRP1 polymorphism was identified as also interacting with STAT4 and IRF5, contributing to disease risk.[42] These studies underline the importance of gene-gene interaction for development of SSc.

GENE EXPRESSION PROFILING

As mentioned, genetics, epigenetics, and gene expression go hand in hand. Gene expression profiling (GEP) in SSc has provided insights into the molecular basis of the disease and the underlying changes that occur during disease progression. Global GEP, which can be performed with microarrays or high-throughput sequencing, allows the simultaneous assessment of thousands of RNA transcripts in a given tissue. It allows examination of gene product interactions along biological pathways.[43] GEP have yielded interesting results that broadened the understanding of SSc. For instance, 2 studies of early diffuse SSc skin gene expression observed differentially expressed genes associated with increased collagen deposition and ECM synthesis.[44–46] One of them analyzed the GEP of affected and unaffected skin (from skin biopsies) as well as fibroblasts from 4 diffuse cutaneous systemic sclerosis (dcSSc) patients and controls (in cultured cells from skin biopsies). More than 2700 genes were differentially expressed between normal and SSc skin biopsies. Interestingly, affected and unaffected skin samples showed nearly identical, disease-specific patterns of gene expression, indicating that the genetic expression in SSc is a systemic process irrespective of clinically appreciated abnormalities. The differences in gene expression were mapped to fibroblasts, epithelial, endothelial, smooth muscle, T and B cells.[45] Taking GEP even further, Assassi and colleagues[47] recently observed that 82 skin transcripts distinguished patients with more severe interstitial lung disease. This list included CCL2 (MCP1), which was also associated with SSc by genetic studies (see **Table 2**). The future of GEP is therefore quite promising because there seems to be a link between gene expression in easily accessible tissues such as skin and internal organ involvement, which not only offers insight into the systemic process and pathophysiology but also could someday aid in risk stratification, prognosis, and treatment decisions.

SUMMARY

The different genetic susceptibility pathways identified so far have offered great insight into the pathophysiology of SSc. The information that has been obtained and that will continue to emerge will provide better disease prognosis and drug responsiveness classification or even predict adverse drug side effects (pharmacogenetics). Discoveries in the field can also lead to identification of novel therapeutic targets and guide drug and biomarker development. As the knowledge of these mechanisms expands, so does the understanding of the intricate pathways necessary to maintain tissue-specific gene expression homeostasis and a healthy state. There is still a big part of the story that remains to be told; the field is evolving daily, offering new insights just around the corner.

REFERENCES

1. Mayes MD, Bossini-Castillo L, Gorlova O, et al. Immunochip analysis identifies multiple susceptibility loci for systemic sclerosis. Am J Hum Genet 2014;94(1):47–61.
2. Agarwal SK. The genetics of systemic sclerosis. Discov Med 2010;10(51):134–43.

3. Granel B, Bernard F, Chevillard C. Genetic susceptibility to systemic sclerosis from clinical aspect to genetic factor analyses. Eur J Intern Med 2009;20(3): 242–52.

4. Allanore Y, Dieude P, Boileau C. Genetic background of systemic sclerosis: auto-immune genes take centre stage. Rheumatology (Oxford) 2010;49(2):203–10.

5. Zhou X, Tan FK, Wang N, et al. Genome-wide association study for regions of systemic sclerosis susceptibility in a Choctaw Indian population with high disease prevalence. Arthritis Rheum 2003;48(9):2585–92.

6. Hudson M, Rojas-Villarraga A, Coral-Alvarado P, et al. Polyautoimmunity and familial autoimmunity in systemic sclerosis. J Autoimmun 2008;31(2):156–9.

7. Martin J, Fonseca C. The genetics of scleroderma. Curr Rheumatol Rep 2011; 13(1):13–20.

8. Mayes MD. The genetics of scleroderma: looking into the postgenomic era. Curr Opin Rheumatol 2012;24(6):677–84.

9. Broen JC, Coenen MJ, Radstake TR. Genetics of systemic sclerosis: an update. Curr Rheumatol Rep 2012;14(1):11–21.

10. Broen JC, Radstake TR, Rossato M. The role of genetics and epigenetics in the pathogenesis of systemic sclerosis. Nat Rev Rheumatol 2014;10(11):671–81.

11. Romano E, Manetti M, Guiducci S, et al. The genetics of systemic sclerosis: an update. Clin Exp Rheumatol 2011;29(2 Suppl 65):S75–86.

12. Assassi S, Radstake TR, Mayes MD, et al. Genetics of scleroderma: implications for personalized medicine? BMC Med 2013;11:9.

13. Radstake TR, Gorlova O, Rueda B, et al. Genome-wide association study of systemic sclerosis identifies CD247 as a new susceptibility locus. Nat Genet 2010; 42(5):426–9.

14. Allanore Y, Saad M, Dieude P, et al. Genome-wide scan identifies TNIP1, PSORS1C1, and RHOB as novel risk loci for systemic sclerosis. PLoS Genet 2011;7(7):e1002091.

15. Martin JE, Bossini-Castillo L, Martin J. Unraveling the genetic component of systemic sclerosis. Hum Genet 2012;131(7):1023–37.

16. Martin JE, Assassi S, Diaz-Gallo LM, et al. A systemic sclerosis and systemic lupus erythematosus pan-meta-GWAS reveals new shared susceptibility loci. Hum Mol Genet 2013;22(19):4021–9.

17. Agarwal SK, Tan FK, Arnett FC. Genetics and genomic studies in scleroderma (systemic sclerosis). Rheum Dis Clin North Am 2008;34(1):17–40.

18. Tan FK, Arnett FC. Genetic factors in the etiology of systemic sclerosis and Raynaud phenomenon. Curr Opin Rheumatol 2000;12(6):511–9.

19. Tan FK. Systemic sclerosis: the susceptible host (genetics and environment). Rheum Dis Clin North Am 2003;29(2):211–37.

20. Arnett FC, Gourh P, Shete S, et al. Major histocompatibility complex (MHC) class II alleles, haplotypes and epitopes which confer susceptibility or protection in systemic sclerosis: analyses in 1300 Caucasian, African-American and Hispanic cases and 1000 controls. Ann Rheum Dis 2010;69(5):822–7.

21. Gorlova O, Martin JE, Rueda B, et al. Identification of novel genetic markers associated with clinical phenotypes of systemic sclerosis through a genome-wide association strategy. PLoS Genet 2011;7(7):e1002178.

22. Reich K, Huffmeier U, Konig IR, et al. TNF polymorphisms in psoriasis: association of psoriatic arthritis with the promoter polymorphism TNF*-857 independent of the PSORS1 risk allele. Arthritis Rheum 2007;56(6):2056–64.

23. Wu M, Assassi S. The role of type 1 interferon in systemic sclerosis. Front Immunol 2013;4:266.

24. Carmona FD, Cenit MC, Diaz-Gallo LM, et al. New insight on the Xq28 association with systemic sclerosis. Ann Rheum Dis 2013;72(12):2032–8.
25. D'Amico F, Skarmoutsou E, Marchini M, et al. Genetic polymorphisms of FOXP3 in Italian patients with systemic sclerosis. Immunol Lett 2013;152(2):109–13.
26. Westra HJ, Franke L. From genome to function by studying eQTLs. Biochim Biophys Acta 2014;1842(10):1896–902.
27. Wittkopp PJ. Genomic sources of regulatory variation in cis and in trans. Cell Mol Life Sci 2005;62(16):1779–83.
28. Bryois J, Buil A, Evans DM, et al. Cis and trans effects of human genomic variants on gene expression. PLoS Genet 2014;10(7):e1004461.
29. Hindorff LA, Sethupathy P, Junkins HA, et al. Potential etiologic and functional implications of genome-wide association loci for human diseases and traits. Proc Natl Acad Sci U S A 2009;106(23):9362–7.
30. De CL, Baralle M, Buratti E. Exon and intron definition in pre-mRNA splicing. Wiley Interdiscip Rev RNA 2013;4(1):49–60.
31. Lewandowska MA. The missing puzzle piece: splicing mutations. Int J Clin Exp Pathol 2013;6(12):2675–82.
32. Seth P, Walker LC, Yeowell HN. Identification of exonic cis-elements regulating the alternative splicing of scleroderma-associated lysyl hydroxylase 2 mRNA. J Invest Dermatol 2011;131(2):537–9.
33. Hulse AM, Cai JJ. Genetic variants contribute to gene expression variability in humans. Genetics 2013;193(1):95–108.
34. Westra HJ, Peters MJ, Esko T, et al. Systematic identification of trans eQTLs as putative drivers of known disease associations. Nat Genet 2013;45(10): 1238–43.
35. van RE. The art of microRNA research. Circ Res 2011;108(2):219–34.
36. Jiang X, Tsitsiou E, Herrick SE, et al. MicroRNAs and the regulation of fibrosis. FEBS J 2010;277(9):2015–21.
37. He Y, Huang C, Lin X, et al. MicroRNA-29 family, a crucial therapeutic target for fibrosis diseases. Biochimie 2013;95(7):1355–9.
38. Vettori S, Gay S, Distler O. Role of MicroRNAs in fibrosis. Open Rheumatol J 2012;6:130–9.
39. Sethupathy P, Megraw M, Hatzigeorgiou AG. A guide through present computational approaches for the identification of mammalian microRNA targets. Nat Methods 2006;3(11):881–6.
40. Imamura K, Akimitsu N. Long non-coding RNAs involved in immune responses. Front Immunol 2014;5:573.
41. Dieude P, Guedj M, Wipff J, et al. STAT4 is a genetic risk factor for systemic sclerosis having additive effects with IRF5 on disease susceptibility and related pulmonary fibrosis. Arthritis Rheum 2009;60(8):2472–9.
42. Dieude P, Wipff J, Guedj M, et al. BANK1 is a genetic risk factor for diffuse cutaneous systemic sclerosis and has additive effects with IRF5 and STAT4. Arthritis Rheum 2009;60(11):3447–54.
43. Assassi S, Mayes MD. What does global gene expression profiling tell us about the pathogenesis of systemic sclerosis? Curr Opin Rheumatol 2013;25(6): 686–91.
44. Sargent JL, Whitfield ML. Capturing the heterogeneity in systemic sclerosis with genome-wide expression profiling. Expert Rev Clin Immunol 2011;7(4):463–73.
45. Whitfield ML, Finlay DR, Murray JI, et al. Systemic and cell type-specific gene expression patterns in scleroderma skin. Proc Natl Acad Sci U S A 2003; 100(21):12319–24.

46. Gardner H, Shearstone JR, Bandaru R, et al. Gene profiling of scleroderma skin reveals robust signatures of disease that are imperfectly reflected in the transcript profiles of explanted fibroblasts. Arthritis Rheum 2006;54(6):1961–73.

47. Assassi S, Wu M, Tan FK, et al. Skin gene expression correlates of severity of interstitial lung disease in systemic sclerosis. Arthritis Rheum 2013;65(11): 2917–27.

48. Sharif R, Mayes MD, Tan FK, et al. IRF5 polymorphism predicts prognosis in patients with systemic sclerosis. Ann Rheum Dis 2012;71(7):1197–202.

49. Dieude P, Guedj M, Wipff J, et al. Association between the IRF5 rs2004640 functional polymorphism and systemic sclerosis: a new perspective for pulmonary fibrosis. Arthritis Rheum 2009;60(1):225–33.

50. Dieude P, Dawidowicz K, Guedj M, et al. Phenotype-haplotype correlation of IRF5 in systemic sclerosis: role of 2 haplotypes in disease severity. J Rheumatol 2010;37(5):987–92.

51. Carmona FD, Martin JE, Beretta L, et al. The systemic lupus erythematosus IRF5 risk haplotype is associated with systemic sclerosis. PLoS One 2013;8(1): e54419.

52. Ito I, Kawaguchi Y, Kawasaki A, et al. Association of a functional polymorphism in the IRF5 region with systemic sclerosis in a Japanese population. Arthritis Rheum 2009;60(6):1845–50.

53. Carmona FD, Gutala R, Simeon CP, et al. Novel identification of the IRF7 region as an anticentromere autoantibody propensity locus in systemic sclerosis. Ann Rheum Dis 2012;71(1):114–9.

54. Dieude P, Guedj M, Wipff J, et al. NLRP1 influences the systemic sclerosis phenotype: a new clue for the contribution of innate immunity in systemic sclerosis-related fibrosing alveolitis pathogenesis. Ann Rheum Dis 2011;70(4): 668–74.

55. Rueda B, Gourh P, Broen J, et al. BANK1 functional variants are associated with susceptibility to diffuse systemic sclerosis in Caucasians. Ann Rheum Dis 2010; 69(4):700–5.

56. Gourh P, Agarwal SK, Martin E, et al. Association of the C8orf13-BLK region with systemic sclerosis in North-American and European populations. J Autoimmun 2010;34(2):155–62.

57. Ito I, Kawaguchi Y, Kawasaki A, et al. Association of the FAM167A-BLK region with systemic sclerosis. Arthritis Rheum 2010;62(3):890–5.

58. Coustet B, Dieude P, Guedj M, et al. C8orf13-BLK is a genetic risk locus for systemic sclerosis and has additive effects with BANK1: results from a large French cohort and meta-analysis. Arthritis Rheum 2011;63(7):2091–6.

59. Dieude P, Bouaziz M, Guedj M, et al. Evidence of the contribution of the X chromosome to systemic sclerosis susceptibility: association with the functional IRAK1 196Phe/532Ser haplotype. Arthritis Rheum 2011;63(12):3979–87.

60. Gourh P, Agarwal SK, Divecha D, et al. Polymorphisms in TBX21 and STAT4 increase the risk of systemic sclerosis: evidence of possible gene-gene interaction and alterations in Th1/Th2 cytokines. Arthritis Rheum 2009;60(12): 3794–806.

61. Rueda B, Broen J, Simeon C, et al. The STAT4 gene influences the genetic predisposition to systemic sclerosis phenotype. Hum Mol Genet 2009;18(11): 2071–7.

62. Tsuchiya N, Kawasaki A, Hasegawa M, et al. Association of STAT4 polymorphism with systemic sclerosis in a Japanese population. Ann Rheum Dis 2009;68(8):1375–6.

63. Dieude P, Boileau C, Guedj M, et al. Independent replication establishes the CD247 gene as a genetic systemic sclerosis susceptibility factor. Ann Rheum Dis 2011;70(9):1695–6.

64. Dieude P, Guedj M, Wipff J, et al. Association of the TNFAIP3 rs5029939 variant with systemic sclerosis in the European Caucasian population. Ann Rheum Dis 2010;69(11):1958–64.

65. Martin JE, Broen JC, Carmona FD, et al. Identification of CSK as a systemic sclerosis genetic risk factor through Genome Wide Association Study follow-up. Hum Mol Genet 2012;21(12):2825–35.

66. Koumakis E, Giraud M, Dieude P, et al. Brief report: candidate gene study in systemic sclerosis identifies a rare and functional variant of the TNFAIP3 locus as a risk factor for polyautoimmunity. Arthritis Rheum 2012;64(8):2746–52.

67. Gourh P, Tan FK, Assassi S, et al. Association of the PTPN22 R620W polymorphism with anti-topoisomerase I- and anticentromere antibody-positive systemic sclerosis. Arthritis Rheum 2006;54(12):3945–53.

68. Dieude P, Guedj M, Wipff J, et al. The PTPN22 620W allele confers susceptibility to systemic sclerosis: findings of a large case-control study of European Caucasians and a meta-analysis. Arthritis Rheum 2008;58(7):2183–8.

69. Diaz-Gallo LM, Gourh P, Broen J, et al. Analysis of the influence of PTPN22 gene polymorphisms in systemic sclerosis. Ann Rheum Dis 2011;70(3):454–62.

70. Gourh P, Arnett FC, Tan FK, et al. Association of TNFSF4 (OX40L) polymorphisms with susceptibility to systemic sclerosis. Ann Rheum Dis 2010;69(3):550–5.

71. Bossini-Castillo L, Broen JC, Simeon CP, et al. A replication study confirms the association of TNFSF4 (OX40L) polymorphisms with systemic sclerosis in a large European cohort. Ann Rheum Dis 2011;70(4):638–41.

72. Coustet B, Bouaziz M, Dieude P, et al. Independent replication and meta analysis of association studies establish TNFSF4 as a susceptibility gene preferentially associated with the subset of anticentromere-positive patients with systemic sclerosis. J Rheumatol 2012;39(5):997–1003.

73. Dieude P, Guedj M, Truchetet ME, et al. Association of the CD226 Ser (307) variant with systemic sclerosis: evidence of a contribution of costimulation pathways in systemic sclerosis pathogenesis. Arthritis Rheum 2011;63(4):1097–105.

74. Bossini-Castillo L, Simeon CP, Beretta L, et al. A multicenter study confirms CD226 gene association with systemic sclerosis-related pulmonary fibrosis. Arthritis Res Ther 2012;14(2):R85.

75. Mattuzzi S, Barbi S, Carletto A, et al. Association of polymorphisms in the IL1B and IL2 genes with susceptibility and severity of systemic sclerosis. J Rheumatol 2007;34(5):997–1004.

76. Martin JE, Carmona FD, Broen JC, et al. The autoimmune disease-associated IL2RA locus is involved in the clinical manifestations of systemic sclerosis. Genes Immun 2012;13(2):191–6.

77. Cenit MC, Simeon CP, Vonk MC, et al. Influence of the IL6 gene in susceptibility to systemic sclerosis. J Rheumatol 2012;39(12):2294–302.

78. Crilly A, Hamilton J, Clark CJ, et al. Analysis of the 5' flanking region of the interleukin 10 gene in patients with systemic sclerosis. Rheumatology (Oxford) 2003;42(11):1295–8.

79. Hudson LL, Rocca KM, Kuwana M, et al. Interleukin-10 genotypes are associated with systemic sclerosis and influence disease-associated autoimmune responses. Genes Immun 2005;6(3):274–8.

80. Bossini-Castillo L, Martin JE, Broen J, et al. A GWAS follow-up study reveals the association of the IL12RB2 gene with systemic sclerosis in Caucasian populations. Hum Mol Genet 2012;21(4):926–33.
81. Granel B, Chevillard C, Allanore Y, et al. Evaluation of interleukin 13 polymorphisms in systemic sclerosis. Immunogenetics 2006;58(8):693–9.
82. Diaz-Gallo LM, Simeon CP, Broen JC, et al. Implication of IL-2/IL-21 region in systemic sclerosis genetic susceptibility. Ann Rheum Dis 2013;72(7):1233–8.
83. Agarwal SK, Gourh P, Shete S, et al. Association of interleukin 23 receptor polymorphisms with anti-topoisomerase-I positivity and pulmonary hypertension in systemic sclerosis. J Rheumatol 2009;36(12):2715–23.
84. Karrer S, Bosserhoff AK, Weiderer P, et al. The -2518 promotor polymorphism in the MCP-1 gene is associated with systemic sclerosis. J Invest Dermatol 2005; 124(1):92–8.
85. Tan FK, Wang N, Kuwana M, et al. Association of fibrillin 1 single-nucleotide polymorphism haplotypes with systemic sclerosis in Choctaw and Japanese populations. Arthritis Rheum 2001;44(4):893–901.
86. Wipff J, Giraud M, Sibilia J, et al. Polymorphic markers of the fibrillin-1 gene and systemic sclerosis in European Caucasian patients. J Rheumatol 2008;35(4):643–9.
87. Fonseca C, Lindahl GE, Ponticos M, et al. A polymorphism in the CTGF promoter region associated with systemic sclerosis. N Engl J Med 2007;357(12): 1210–20.
88. Zhou X, Tan FK, Reveille JD, et al. Association of novel polymorphisms with the expression of SPARC in normal fibroblasts and with susceptibility to scleroderma. Arthritis Rheum 2002;46(11):2990–9.
89. Makino K, Jinnin M, Hirano A, et al. The downregulation of microRNA let-7a contributes to the excessive expression of type I collagen in systemic and localized scleroderma. J Immunol 2013;190(8):3905–15.
90. Zhu H, Li Y, Qu S, et al. MicroRNA expression abnormalities in limited cutaneous scleroderma and diffuse cutaneous scleroderma. J Clin Immunol 2012;32(3): 514–22.
91. Maurer B, Stanczyk J, Jungel A, et al. MicroRNA-29, a key regulator of collagen expression in systemic sclerosis. Arthritis Rheum 2010;62(6):1733–43.
92. Takemoto R, Jinnin M, Wang Z, et al. Hair miR-29a levels are decreased in patients with scleroderma. Exp Dermatol 2013;22(12):832–3.
93. Tanaka S, Suto A, Ikeda K, et al. Alteration of circulating miRNAs in SSc: miR-30b regulates the expression of PDGF receptor beta. Rheumatology (Oxford) 2013;52(11):1963–72.
94. Li H, Yang R, Fan X, et al. MicroRNA array analysis of microRNAs related to systemic scleroderma. Rheumatol Int 2012;32(2):307–13.
95. Nakashima T, Jinnin M, Yamane K, et al. Impaired IL-17 signaling pathway contributes to the increased collagen expression in scleroderma fibroblasts. J Immunol 2012;188(8):3573–83.
96. Honda N, Jinnin M, Kira-Etoh T, et al. miR-150 down-regulation contributes to the constitutive type I collagen overexpression in scleroderma dermal fibroblasts via the induction of integrin β3. Am J Pathol 2013;182(1):206–16.
97. Honda N, Jinnin M, Kajihara I, et al. TGF-β-mediated downregulation of microRNA-196a contributes to the constitutive upregulated type I collagen expression in scleroderma dermal fibroblasts. J Immunol 2012;188(7):3323–31.
98. Wang Z, Jinnin M, Kudo H, et al. Detection of hair-microRNAs as the novel potent biomarker: evaluation of the usefulness for the diagnosis of scleroderma. J Dermatol Sci 2013;72(2):134–41.

99. Makino K, Jinnin M, Aoi J, et al. Discoidin domain receptor 2-microRNA 196a-mediated negative feedback against excess type I collagen expression is impaired in scleroderma dermal fibroblasts. J Invest Dermatol 2013;133(1): 110–9.

100. Kajihara I, Jinnin M, Yamane K, et al. Increased accumulation of extracellular thrombospondin-2 due to low degradation activity stimulates type I collagen expression in scleroderma fibroblasts. Am J Pathol 2012;180(2):703–14.

101. Zhu H, Luo H, Li Y, et al. MicroRNA-21 in scleroderma fibrosis and its function in TGF-β-regulated fibrosis-related genes expression. J Clin Immunol 2013;33(6): 1100–9.

102. Sing T, Jinnin M, Yamane K, et al. microRNA-92a expression in the sera and dermal fibroblasts increases in patients with scleroderma. Rheumatology (Oxford) 2012;51(9):1550–6.

103. Makino K, Jinnin M, Kajihara I, et al. Circulating miR-142-3p levels in patients with systemic sclerosis. Clin Exp Dermatol 2012;37(1):34–9.

The Pathogenesis of Systemic Sclerosis

Edward P. Stern, MBBS, MRCP, Christopher P. Denton, PhD, FRCP*

KEYWORDS

- Systemic sclerosis • Scleroderma • Pathogenesis • Fibrosis • Autoimmunity
- Vasculopathy

KEY POINTS

- Systemic sclerosis is a multisystem disorder with a high associated mortality.
- The hallmark abnormalities of the disease are in the immune system, vasculature, and connective tissue.
- Systemic sclerosis occurs in susceptible individuals (as defined by genetic studies) and is stimulated by initiating events, although these initiating factors are poorly understood at present.
- In order for the disease phenotype to appear there is dysfunction in the homoeostatic mechanisms of immune tolerance, endothelial physiology, and extracellular matrix turnover.
- The progression of disease is not sequential but requires simultaneous dysfunction in these normal regulatory mechanisms.
- A better understanding of the interplay of these factors is likely to contribute to improved treatment options.

INTRODUCTION

Systemic sclerosis (SSc; also called scleroderma) is a complex multisystem disorder with heterogeneous clinical features. The disease is broadly divided by clinical phenotypes, which include limited cutaneous and diffuse cutaneous SSc (dcSSc). Almost all individuals with SSc have detectable circulating antibodies against nuclear proteins and different SSc phenotypes are strongly associated with the different antibody types. However, in most cases the recognized antibodies are not directly disease causing. To date there is only limited evidence as to the primary causes of SSc and the molecular phenomena underlying its clinical features. It is to be hoped that, by

Disclosures: None.
Centre for Rheumatology, UCL Royal Free Campus, Rowland Hill Street, London NW3 2PF, UK
* Corresponding author.
E-mail address: c.denton@ucl.ac.uk

Rheum Dis Clin N Am 41 (2015) 367–382
http://dx.doi.org/10.1016/j.rdc.2015.04.002
0889-857X/15/$ – see front matter © 2015 Elsevier Inc. All rights reserved.

achieving a fuller understanding of the pathogenesis of this disease, the management options for affected individuals will be improved and the associated burden of morbidity and mortality reduced.

The SSc phenotype includes demonstrable abnormalities in the immune, connective tissue, and vascular systems of affected individuals. There have been many important observations regarding the role of dysregulation in these 3 systems and interplay between the systems in the SSc disease process and this article summarizes some of the key findings. In addition, investigations into the genetic background of patients with scleroderma have allowed clinicians to perceive this as a disease that occurs when a susceptible individual is exposed to particular environmental factors, and the molecular processes are treated here in this broader context. As well as these unifying observations about the disease processes, a convincing account of the pathogenesis of SSc needs to account for the heterogeneity of its clinical presentations.

Overview of Etiopathogenesis

One of the hallmarks of SSc is the interplay between vascular damage, inflammation, and connective tissue repair and this led to models of pathogenesis that were often linear, suggesting that immune or inflammatory events followed minor vascular injury and led to fibrosis and scarring. This paradigm does not fit well with clinical observations of disease heterogeneity and the differential involvement and progression in individual organ systems. A more integrated model sees all of these processes as being relevant as the disease develops, progresses, and potentially improves in later stages. Thus it is more relevant to consider processes that reflect or contribute to early initiation or triggering, amplification, and later progression of SSc. The relationship between these stages in etiopathogenesis is summarized in **Fig. 1**.

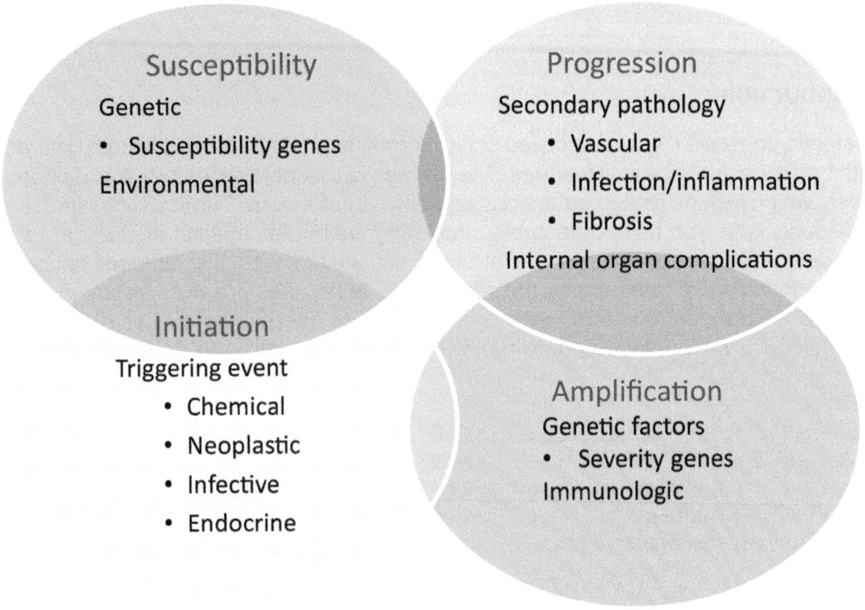

Susceptibility
Genetic
- Susceptibility genes
Environmental

Progression
Secondary pathology
- Vascular
- Infection/inflammation
- Fibrosis
Internal organ complications

Initiation
Triggering event
- Chemical
- Neoplastic
- Infective
- Endocrine

Amplification
Genetic factors
- Severity genes
Immunologic

Fig. 1. Etiopathogenesis of SSC.

SUSCEPTIBILITY
Epidemiology

Epidemiologic studies have shown a significant increase in the risk of SSc in first-degree relatives of patients with the disease: 1.6% versus a 0.026% risk in the general population,[1] and there is strong evidence of familial clustering of cases. In these clusters, relatives tend to have the same disease-associated autoantibody.[1,2] These data imply a genetic susceptibility to SSc overall and an inherited susceptibility to develop the specific subgroups of disease.

Human Leukocyte Antigen Associations

Like other autoimmune rheumatic diseases, scleroderma is consistently associated with polymorphisms in the human leukocyte antigen (HLA) region of the major histocompatibility complex. Modest associations have been seen between given haplotypes and the disease overall.[3,4] Stronger specific HLA associations have been shown for each of the major autoantibody subgroups of scleroderma; for example, HLA DQB1-0501 is associated with the anticentromere antibody (ACA),[5] and DRB1*1104 and DPB1*1301 are both independently associated with the anti–topoisomerase I antibody (ATA).[6,7]

Candidate Gene Studies

In addition to these HLA associations, candidate gene studies have shown associations with polymorphisms in genes relevant to the 3 key "compartments" of SSc: the immune, connective tissue, and vascular systems.

Positive associations with polymorphisms found in candidate genes governing vascular function have included endothelial nitric oxide synthase (eNOS), angiotensin-converting enzyme (ACE),[8] and the endothelin receptor (ETR) B.[9] Disease-associated polymorphisms in genes involved in the connective tissue system include connective tissue growth factor (CTGF),[10] fibrillin-1[11] and secreted protein acidic and rich in cysteine (SPARC).[12] However, none of these associations have been replicated across multiple populations.

In contrast, positive candidate gene studies examining associations with genetic loci regulating the immune system have been successfully replicated. These genes include STAT4, an important regulator of T-cell differentiation[13]; BANK1, a regulator of B-cell activation[14]; and IRF5, an activator of type 1 interferon.[15] Some of these target genes have specific associations with particular organ complications of SSc; for instance, STAT4 polymorphisms and pulmonary fibrosis.[16]

Genome-wide Association Studies

Large genome-wide association studies (GWAS) in North America, Europe, and east Asia, including several thousand patients with SSc in total, have confirmed some of the associations seen in candidate gene studies, including those with STAT4[17] and IRF5.[18] The best-replicated susceptibility gene newly identified via GWAS has been CD247, a mediator of T-cell receptor signaling, previously seen to be involved in the pathogenesis of systemic lupus erythematosus (SLE).[17,19]

Further GWAS analysis has successfully identified loci associated with phenotypic (limited vs diffuse SSc) and immunologic (ACA vs ATA) subgroups of SSc.[20] Given the well-described associations between disease subgroups, antibodies, and disease complications, there is an opportunity for future GWAS analysis to examine extreme phenotypes of SSc that include antibody, skin phenotype, and internal organ complications. For example, Guerra et al [21] identified genetic loci that differentiated between patients who were renal crisis positive and renal crisis negative within a cohort of patients with both dcSSc and the RNA polymerase III antibody (ARA). This study confirmed previously seen associations with HLA and complement regions and suggested additional candidate loci that are now being further investigated. Genetic associations for SSc are summarized in **Table 1**.

INITIATION
Chemical Triggers

The syndrome of Raynaud phenomenon, skin thickening, and acro-osteolysis seen with occupational exposure to vinyl chloride was first recognized in the 1960s[22] and is markedly similar to SSc in many respects. The HLA antigens predicting development and severity of vinyl chloride disease mirror those that are predictive in SSc.[23,24] This finding exemplifies the concept of SSc as a disease initiated by one or more exposure factors in a susceptible individual. Other chemical agents that have been observed to cause scleroderma-like clinical features include taxane chemotherapy,[25] contaminated rapeseed oil,[26] and tryptophan.[27]

Following on from this hypothesis, in the broader population of patients with a diagnosis of SSc, several environmental factors have been investigated as risks for development of the disease. The best-recognized association is between exposure to solvents in the workplace and the risk of SSc.[28,29] This increased risk seems to be more marked in men, regardless of exposure dose,[30] supporting the hypothesis that exposure risks are acquired in the context of a variable degree of genetic susceptibility. Other strong occupational risk factors for SSc, including crystalline silica and white spirit, also show this marked gender difference in the additional risk conferred.[29]

Table 1		
Non-HLA genes associated with an increased risk of the incidence of SSC		
Pathogenic Association	**Gene**	**Study Type**
Vascular	eNOS	Candidate gene
	ACE	Candidate gene
	ET-1	Candidate gene
	ETR-A/B	Candidate gene
Immune/inflammation	STAT4	Candidate gene/GWAS[a]
	IRF5	Candidate gene/GWAS[a]
	CD247	GWAS[a]
	TNIP1	GWAS[a]
	BLK	Candidate gene[a]
	TNFSF4	Candidate gene[a]
	BANK1	Candidate gene[a]
	MIF	Candidate gene[a]
Connective tissue	CTGF	Candidate gene
	Fibrillin-1	Candidate gene
	SPARC	Candidate gene

Abbreviations: BANK1, B call scaffold protein with ankyrin repeats 1; BLK, B lymphocyte kinase; CD247, cluster of differentiation 247; ET-1, endothelin-1; IRF5, interferon regulatory factor 5; MIF, macrophage migration inhibitory factor; STAT4, signal transducer and activator of transcription 4; TNFSF4, tumor necrosis factor superfamily 4; TNIP1, TNFAIP3 (tumor necrosis factor, alpha-induced protein 3) interacting protein 1.
[a] The association of these genes has been replicated across more than 1 population study.

Endocrine Triggers

Several hypotheses have attempted to account for the increased prevalence of SSc and other autoimmune disease in women (around 5:1 for SSc). There is some evidence that endocrine triggers may be involved in the initiation or propagation of the disease state. In particular, it has been noted that the female sex hormone estradiol increases the profibrotic effects of some important mediators of SSc (interferon-gamma, interleukin [IL]-1, and tumor necrosis factor alpha).[31]

Infective Triggers

As in other autoimmune diseases, it has been postulated that SSc is triggered in at least some individuals via a host immune response to an infective agent that is a molecular mimic for self-proteins. For example, it has been observed that there are close resemblances in amino acid sequences between the ATA antigen and a group-specific antigen on some mammalian retroviruses.[32]

A more specific hypothesis regarding infective triggering for scleroderma concerns the role of latent cytomegalovirus (CMV) infection, which can localize to the endothelium. To support this putative relationship, potentially pathogenic autoantigens seen in SSc bind to the UL94 protein on CMV and also to the human endothelial cell surface, where they cause endothelial apoptosis (endothelial cell injury is traditionally considered an early event in the SSc disease process, as discussed later).[33]

Neoplastic Triggers

One setting in which the onset of SSc in relation to a trigger has been well delineated on a molecular level is in the subgroup of patients with SSc and cancer. It has been observed that there is a high incidence of malignancy in patients with scleroderma and the ARA antibody and that, in this subgroup, the onset of connective tissue disease and cancer diagnosis have a close temporal relationship.[34,35] Joseph and colleagues[36] identified alterations in the RNA polymerase III polypeptide A gene (POL3RA) in neoplastic cells extracted from tumors of patients in this subgroup, but not in control tissues from the same patients or in the tumor tissues of patients from other scleroderma subgroups. The investigators hypothesized that highly specific cellular immunity triggered by a neoplastic mutation could lose its specificity in the humoral response (epitope spreading) and that this sequence of events could produce an autoimmune phenotype. To support this, they identified a population of CD4 T cells in the peripheral blood of some of these patients that were specifically reactive to the mutant POL3RA alleles in their tumor tissue (but not to the wild type) and showed that the humoral (antibody) response in these patients did not discriminate between wild-type and mutant POL3RA.

This study provides a helpfully detailed example of how an autoimmune disease such as SSc might be triggered in a susceptible individual by exposure to a cross-reactive antigen (in this case a somatic mutation in tumor tissue).

PROGRESSION

The most-commonly postulated model of disease progression in SSc is sequential, with immune activation and subsequent vasculopathy leading to activation of fibroblasts and fibrosis as the end effect of these processes.[37] However, it is not proven in what order these events take place. It seems that the disease state is only tolerated if there is simultaneous dysregulation of the immune system, vascular endothelium, and connective tissue repair system. It is in the context of the disease susceptibility and initiation discussed earlier that the cardinal features of scleroderma (fibrosis of

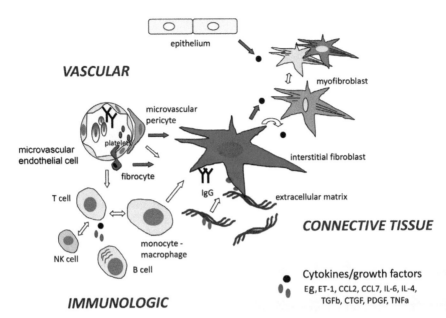

Fig. 2. Cellular interplay in the pathogenesis of SSc. CCL2, chemokine ligand 2; CCL7, chemokine ligand 7; CTGF, connective tissue growth factor; ET-1, endothelin-1; IgG, immunoglobulin G; NK, natural killer; PDGF, platelet-derived growth factor; TGFb, transforming growth factor beta; TNFa, tumor necrosis factor alpha.

the skin and internal organs and systemic vasculopathy) are allowed to develop and are subsequently amplified. The interplay of cell types and signaling molecules implicated in the disease state is summarized in **Fig. 2**.

Raynaud Phenomenon and the Role of Vasoconstrictors

Alterations in the cells and physiologic activity of the vascular endothelium seem to be of especial importance in the pathophysiology of SSc.[38] Within this, mediators of vascular tone, including the endothelins and nitric oxide, play a key role.[39]

Endothelin-1 (ET-1), a uniquely potent vasoconstrictor and also a mediator of fibrosis,[40] has been proposed to be an important effector molecule in SSc. ET-1 levels have been shown to be dynamically responsive to cold in patients with SSc with Raynaud phenomenon but not in healthy controls.[41] ET-1 was also shown to promote collagen synthesis in a dose-dependent manner in these patients. Circulating ET-1 levels have been found to correlate with both disease severity and the progression of important disease complications, including pulmonary arterial hypertension, interstitial lung disease, and scleroderma renal crisis (SRC).[42–44] Both ETR-A and ETR-B have been shown to be overexpressed in affected tissues in SRC.[45]

As both a dynamic regulator of vascular tone and an effector molecule in fibrosis, ET-1 seems to play a linking and promoting role between these systems in SSc: staining for ET-1 and for the endothelin receptor were increased in the vasculature and superficial dermis of patients with scleroderma with both uninvolved skin and early skin fibrosis but not in skin showing late fibrosis.[46]

In clinical care, pharmacologic antagonists of ETR-A and ETR-B have proved to be effective clinical treatments for apparently diverse vasculopathic complications of SSc (digital ulceration and pulmonary arterial hypertension). This finding provides further evidence that the endothelin system plays a significant part in the disease process.

Outside of the disease state, endothelin system activity is regulated by direct negative feedback (via ETR-B) and also by nitric oxide synthase and superoxide anions. It is likely that some or all of these homeostatic mechanisms are defective in SSc, but evidence regarding the specific defects is contradictory.[47–49]

Endothelial Damage in Systemic Sclerosis

Anti–endothelial cell antibodies have been detected in the sera of a significant minority of patients with scleroderma and the sera of these patients has been shown in vitro to induce endothelial cell apoptosis.[50–52] In some cases this apoptosis has been able to be blocked by anti–tumor necrosis factor antibodies. The complement membrane attack complex has been shown in the microvasculature of affected tissues in SSc.[53] After endothelial damage, increased shear stresses and reperfusion injury are both likely to play a role in the progression of SSc vasculopathy.[54,55] Vascular repair and angiogenesis are observed to be defective in SSc, promoting the chronic disease state.[56,57]

Adhesion Molecules

Adhesion molecules, which mediate interactions between the vasculature and extracellular matrix and regulate the migration of lymphocytes, seem to have a significant role in the pathologic processes of SSc.[58,59] Expression of the intercellular adhesion molecule-1 (ICAM-1) and endothelial leukocyte adhesion molecule-1 (E-selectin) on the endothelial cell surface have been shown to be increased in patients with scleroderma.[60]

Furthermore, increased circulating levels of the soluble forms of ICAM-1, E-selectin, and vascular cell adhesion molecule-1 have been shown in the sera of patients with SSc.[48,61,62] Increases in the levels of these 3 soluble adhesion molecules have also been shown to be associated with renal crisis.[63]

Immunologic Activity in Systemic Sclerosis

As discussed earlier, the best-replicated genetic risks for SSc are either in HLA alleles common to other autoimmune diseases or in genes that govern lymphocyte activity. Furthermore, the triggering events reviewed here are presumed to be mediated via the immune system. These findings imply that the immunologic abnormalities seen in the disease have a primary importance in its pathogenesis. However, immunosuppressive medications, although important in the management of SSc, have only had a modest effect on patient outcomes compared with the effectiveness of these agents in rheumatoid arthritis or SLE, which are comparable autoimmune diseases in many respects. For this reason, it is necessary to consider immune abnormalities in the SSc disease state as phenomena that happen in concert with dysfunction in the vasculature and extracellular matrix rather than as a reversible cause of these dysfunctions.

The Role of Autoantibodies

Around 95% of patients with SSc have detectable autoantibodies, which in most cases are highly specific for the disease. The target antigens for the commonly seen antibodies are all intranuclear: the centromere (ACA), topoisomerase 1 (ATA; formerly known as Scl-70), RNA polymerase III antibody (ARA), ribonucleoproteins (fibrillarin or U3RNP), and the exosome complex (Pm-Scl).

Environmental or neoplastic exposures that are thought to provoke antibody production in some cases are discussed earlier. However, in most cases the provocation is not clear, but there is evidence that, in at least some cases, antibody production could be secondary to vasculopathy; it has been shown that several of the scleroderma-associated autoantigens are fragmented by reactive oxygen species

(ROS) in the setting of ischemia-reperfusion injury.[64] The hypothesis is that this fragmentation produces immunogenic peptides that are capable of breaking self-tolerance.

In general, the diagnostic immunoglobulin G antibodies seen in SSc are unlikely to be directly pathogenic, but instead reflect T-cell activity against their antigenic targets. However, circulating antibodies against other targets may be directly implicated in the disease process. As well as antiendothelial antibodies (described earlier), antifibroblast antibodies have been detected in the sera of patients with SSc but not in controls and have been shown in vitro to activate fibroblasts when they react with cell surface molecules.[65] Biologically active anti–angiotensin receptor and anti–endothelin receptor antibodies are also highly prevalent in patients with SSc compared with controls and levels of both antibodies showed a positive correlation with disease severity.[66] A further study found antibodies against the platelet-derived growth factor receptor (PDGFR) to be a specific hallmark of patients with SSc compared with controls. The anti-PDGFR antibodies were shown to generate ROS and stimulate myofibroblast differentiation and type 1 collagen gene expression.[67] None of the studies discussed earlier identify how these apparently pathogenic antibodies are acquired or propagated in SSc.

Cellular Immunity

In the context of the increased cell adhesion molecule activity discussed earlier, migration and activation of CD4-positive T cells is enhanced in SSc[68] and this cell type predominates in the lymphocytic infiltrates seen in both skin and lung tissue.[69,70] Differentiation of the T helper 17 cells (Th17) subclass of T cells may be an important process in SSc and these cells are profibrotic.[71] It has also been proposed that regulatory T cells, which should maintain self-tolerance, are either defective or reduced in number in SSc.[72,73] Monocyte infiltration has also been shown in the skin and lungs of patients and this is potentially mediated by altered function of toll-like receptors.[74,75]

Cytokines and Cell Signaling in Systemic Sclerosis

The paracrine factors important in SSc are not restricted to those stimulated or released by lymphocytes. Endothelial cells and fibroblasts also contribute to the important signaling cascades and appreciating abnormalities in the communication between these 3 cell types will be a vital part of understanding the disease process.

This is a multidirectional interaction. For example, the increased expression of ICAM-1 (discussed earlier), occurring in soluble form and on the surface of both fibroblasts and endothelial cells, increases the binding of lymphocytes to fibroblasts and the transmigration of lymphocytes across the endothelium. The increased ICAM-1 levels have been shown to be stimulated by interferon-gamma and tumor necrosis factor, originating in turn from lymphocytes.[31,76]

In the analysis of this crosstalk between the immune, vascular, and connective tissue systems, a great deal of interest has been concentrated on the signaling mechanisms that promote activation of fibroblasts and/or epithelial-to-mesenchymal transformation, to provide the population of myofibroblasts typical of SSc.

Transforming Growth Factor Beta

A potent stimulator of extracellular matrix production, transforming growth factor (TGF)-beta, has been intensively investigated as a pathogenic mediator in SSc. It is upregulated in affected tissues in the disease[77,78] but circulating TGF-beta has been seen to be reduced in the sera of patients compared with controls, and the levels are inversely correlated with disease activity,[79] suggesting that there could be an increase in binding sites or sequestration of the growth factor in the disease state. TGF-beta receptors have been shown to be upregulated in the skin of patients with SSc compared with controls.[80] However, attempts to induce or maintain a scleroderma-like phenotype in cell culture via manipulation of the TGF-beta system have not been successful.[81]

It is likely that TGF-beta exerts its fibrogenic effects in SSc via other cytokines, including ET-1 and platelet-derived growth factor (PDGF). TGF-beta induces mitosis in fibroblasts acting via the PDGFR. In culture, PDGFR expression in response to TGF-beta from SSc fibroblasts is greatly increased compared with control cells, and the mitogenic response to PDGF is also increased.[82]

Connective Tissue Growth Factor (or CCN2)

CTGF is an important effector in the TGF-beta pathway and its expression is increased in many fibrotic diseases.[83] SSc fibroblasts produce increased levels of CTGF and levels of the N-terminal fragment were increased in dermal blister fluid and in blood from patients and correlated with disease activity.[84] Rather than simply being a downstream effector of TGF-beta, it now seems likely that CTGF is a necessary cofactor for it to activate or sustain extracellular matrix (ECM) production in both healthy and disease states.[85]

Interleukins and Chemokines

IL-6 is a stimulator of collagen synthesis.[86] Levels of this cytokine are increased in patients with scleroderma and correlate with severity of skin involvement.[87] Because IL-6 is secreted by both fibroblasts and lymphocytes, its specific role in the disease process is not clear.

Similarly, IL-4 (predominantly produced by Th2 T-helper cells) is overexpressed in blood and affected tissues in SSc,[88,89] SSc fibroblasts overexpress its receptor, and stimulation of the IL-4 receptor in SSc fibroblasts increases collagen production.[90]

IL-1-alpha secretion from keratinocytes in the epidermis is increased in SSc and coculture of SSc keratinocytes with normal skin fibroblasts caused fibroblast activation, myofibroblast differentiation, and CTGF expression, all mediated by IL-1-alpha.[91]

CXCL4 (or platelet-activating factor 4), an angiogenic factor, downregulates the expression of antifibrotic cytokines (interferon-gamma) and upregulates profibrotic cytokines (IL-4, IL-13).[92] Plasma levels of CXCL4 are increased in SSc and correlate with several measures of disease severity.[93]

Monocyte chemotactic protein (MCP)-1 and MCP-3 are both overexpressed in the disease state.[90,94] MCP-1 in particular may have a directly pathogenic role but both of these proteins, like those listed earlier, are better established as biomarkers of disease activity than as effectors of the disease.

Fibroblasts

The skin and internal organ fibrosis that is pathognomonic in scleroderma depends on the development of a population of activated fibroblasts that produce excess collagen. In cell culture, SSc fibroblasts from both skin and lung show these features compared with normal cells and maintain the phenotype through multiple passages.[95] In vivo, the cells with this phenotype localize to the perivascular tissues and in areas of inflammatory infiltrate, whereas fibroblasts of a normal phenotype persist in other areas.[96,97] It is not clear to what extent the phenotype of increased matrix production is initiated and sustained by an excess of profibrotic signals like those cytokines and growth factors described earlier, or how much this pathophysiology depends on an absence of required inhibitory signals. In normal physiology, matrix production is inhibited when the fibroblast comes into contact with ECM components, including collagen and fibronectin.

The extent to which the fibroblast depends on TGF-beta for sustained ECM production has been examined in animal models in which the TGF-beta receptor gene is deleted. Such transgenic mice were unable to achieve normal wound healing[98] and were resistant to bleomycin-induced lung fibrosis.[99] However, unlike the connective tissue system shown in these models, in vitro experiments imply that the human SSc fibroblast has a degree of autonomy in ECM production without an absolute requirement for external signaling stimuli.[100]

What modifications the cells or their environment have undergone to allow this sustained phenotype is a topic of some debate. It may be that a part of the immune dysfunction of SSc is to select out a population of fibroblasts capable of sustained overproduction of collagen. Another hypothesis is of epigenetic modulation of the cells' activity: in one experiment hypermethylation of the promoter region for the FLI 1 gene (an inhibitor of collagen synthesis) produced a phenotype of stable, ongoing excess collagen production from fibroblasts.[101]

A further possibility is that the fibroblast's activity is modulated by its immediate environment, in particular where the ECM contents are abnormal. One suggestion is that microfibrils of fibrillin-1 in SSc may be more unstable than in normal individuals and that this alters the fibroblast phenotype in a sustained manner.[102,103]

AMPLIFICATION

Up to this point this article describes multiple factors that make an individual susceptible to SSc, including events and exposures that may be responsible for triggering the disease in such an individual. We have also summarized the dysfunctional molecular activity that allows the disease to progress to the extent that the recognizable scleroderma phenotype is seen in patients.

These molecular processes of simultaneous multisystem dysregulation permit the amplification of the disease over time and the specific organ complications that cause the significant morbidity and mortality in SSc. However, genetic factors may at least partially account for the severity of an individual's disease, the phenotypic subgroup, and the risk of developing specific complications of the disease.

FUTURE CONSIDERATIONS

The complex interrelation between the immunologic, vascular, and fibrotic elements of SSc is so far incompletely described. A better understanding of the key processes, in particular those initiating endothelial dysfunction and excessive collagen synthesis, may allow the identification of molecular targets for improved therapies.

REFERENCES

1. Agarwal SK, Tan FK, Arnett FC. Genetics and genomic studies in scleroderma (systemic sclerosis). Rheum Dis Clin North Am 2008;34:17–40, v.
2. Feghali-Bostwick C, Medsger TA, Wright TM. Analysis of systemic sclerosis in twins reveals low concordance for disease and high concordance for the presence of antinuclear antibodies. Arthritis Rheum 2003;48:1956–63.
3. Tan FK, Arnett FC. Genetic factors in the etiology of systemic sclerosis and Raynaud phenomenon. Curr Opin Rheumatol 2000;12:511–9.

4. Tan FK. Systemic sclerosis: the susceptible host (genetics and environment). Rheum Dis Clin North Am 2003;29:211–37.

5. Morel PA, Chang HJ, Wilson JW, et al. HLA and ethnic associations among systemic sclerosis patients with anticentromere antibodies. Hum Immunol 1995;42: 35–42.

6. Reveille JD, Durban E, MacLeod-St Clair MJ, et al. Association of amino acid sequences in the HLA-DQB1 first domain with antitopoisomerase I autoantibody response in scleroderma (progressive systemic sclerosis). J Clin Invest 1992; 90:973–80.

7. Gilchrist FC, Bunn C, Foley PJ, et al. Class II HLA associations with autoantibodies in scleroderma: a highly significant role for HLA-DP. Genes Immun 2001;2:76–81.

8. Fatini C, Gensini F, Sticchi E, et al. High prevalence of polymorphisms of angiotensin-converting enzyme (I/D) and endothelial nitric oxide synthase (Glu298Asp) in patients with systemic sclerosis. Am J Med 2002;112:540–4.

9. Fonseca C, Renzoni E, Sestini P, et al. Endothelin axis polymorphisms in patients with scleroderma. Arthritis Rheum 2006;54:3034–42.

10. Fonseca C, Lindahl GE, Ponticos M, et al. A polymorphism in the CTGF promoter region associated with systemic sclerosis. N Engl J Med 2007;357:1210–20.

11. Tan FK, Stivers DN, Foster MW, et al. Association of microsatellite markers near the fibrillin 1 gene on human chromosome 15q with scleroderma in a Native American population. Arthritis Rheum 1998;41:1729–37.

12. Zhou X, Tan FK, Reveille JD, et al. Association of novel polymorphisms with the expression of SPARC in normal fibroblasts and with susceptibility to scleroderma. Arthritis Rheum 2002;46:2990–9.

13. Rueda B, Broen J, Simeon C, et al. The STAT4 gene influences the genetic predisposition to systemic sclerosis phenotype. Hum Mol Genet 2009;18:2071–7.

14. Rueda B, Gourh P, Broen J, et al. BANK1 functional variants are associated with susceptibility to diffuse systemic sclerosis in Caucasians. Ann Rheum Dis 2010; 69:700–5.

15. Dieudé P, Guedj M, Wipff J, et al. Association between the IRF5 rs2004640 functional polymorphism and systemic sclerosis: a new perspective for pulmonary fibrosis. Arthritis Rheum 2009;60:225–33.

16. Dieudé P, Guedj M, Wipff J, et al. STAT4 is a genetic risk factor for systemic sclerosis having additive effects with IRF5 on disease susceptibility and related pulmonary fibrosis. Arthritis Rheum 2009;60:2472–9.

17. Radstake TR, Gorlova O, Rueda B, et al. Genome-wide association study of systemic sclerosis identifies CD247 as a new susceptibility locus. Nat. Genet. 2010; 42:426–9.

18. Allanore Y, Saad M, Dieudé P, et al. Genome-wide scan identifies TNIP1, PSORS1C1, and RHOB as novel risk loci for systemic sclerosis. PLoS Genet 2011;7:e1002091.

19. Gorman CL, Russell AI, Zhang Z, et al. Polymorphisms in the CD3Z gene influence TCRzeta expression in systemic lupus erythematosus patients and healthy controls. J. Immunol 2008;180:1060–70.

20. Gorlova O, Martin JE, Rueda B, et al. Identification of novel genetic markers associated with clinical phenotypes of systemic sclerosis through a genome-wide association strategy. PLoS Genet 2011;7:e1002178.

21. Guerra SG, Fonseca C, Nihtyanova SI, et al. Defining Genetic Risk for Scleroderma Renal Crisis: A Genome-Wide Analysis of Anti-Rna Polymerase Antibody-Positive Systemic Sclerosis. Br Soc Rheumatol 2015;54(Suppl 1):i159.

22. Binns CH. Vinyl chloride: a review. J Soc Occup Med 1979;29:134–41.
23. Black CM, Welsh KI, Walker AE, et al. Genetic susceptibility to scleroderma-like syndrome induced by vinyl chloride. Lancet 1983;1:53–5.
24. Black C, Pereira S, McWhirter A, et al. Genetic susceptibility to scleroderma-like syndrome in symptomatic and asymptomatic workers exposed to vinyl chloride. J Rheumatol 1986;13:1059–62.
25. Itoh M, Yanaba K, Kobayashi T, et al. Taxane-induced scleroderma. Br J Dermatol 2007;156:363–7.
26. Tabuenca JM. Toxic-allergic syndrome caused by ingestion of rapeseed oil denatured with aniline. Lancet 1981;2:567–8.
27. Silver RM, Heyes MP, Maize JC, et al. Scleroderma, fasciitis, and eosinophilia associated with the ingestion of tryptophan. N Engl J Med 1990;322:874–81.
28. Nietert PJ, Sutherland SE, Silver RM, et al. Is occupational organic solvent exposure a risk factor for scleroderma? Arthritis Rheum 1998;41:1111–8.
29. Marie I, Gehanno JF, Bubenheim M, et al. Prospective study to evaluate the association between systemic sclerosis and occupational exposure and review of the literature. Autoimmun Rev 2014;13:151–6.
30. Kettaneh A, Al Moufti O, Tiev KP, et al. Occupational exposure to solvents and gender-related risk of systemic sclerosis: a metaanalysis of case-control studies. J Rheumatol 2007;34:97–103.
31. Shi-Wen X, Panesar M, Vancheeswaran R, et al. Expression and shedding of intercellular adhesion molecule 1 and lymphocyte function-associated antigen 3 by normal and scleroderma fibroblasts. Effects of interferon-gamma, tumor necrosis factor alpha, and estrogen. Arthritis Rheum 1994;37:1689–97.
32. Maul GG, Jimenez SA, Riggs E, et al. Determination of an epitope of the diffuse systemic sclerosis marker antigen DNA topoisomerase I: sequence similarity with retroviral p30gag protein suggests a possible cause for autoimmunity in systemic sclerosis. Proc Natl Acad Sci U S A 1989;86:8492–6.
33. Lunardi C, Bason C, Navone R, et al. Systemic sclerosis immunoglobulin G autoantibodies bind the human cytomegalovirus late protein UL94 and induce apoptosis in human endothelial cells. Nat Med 2000;6:1183–6.
34. Shah AA, Rosen A, Hummers L, et al. Close temporal relationship between onset of cancer and scleroderma in patients with RNA polymerase I/III antibodies. Arthritis Rheum 2010;62:2787–95.
35. Moinzadeh P, Fonseca C, Hellmich M, et al. Association of anti-RNA polymerase III autoantibodies and cancer in scleroderma. Arthritis Res Ther 2014;16:R53.
36. Joseph CG, Darrah E, Shah AA, et al. Association of the autoimmune disease scleroderma with an immunologic response to cancer. Science 2014;343:152–7.
37. Systemic sclerosis: current pathogenetic concepts and future prospects for targeted therapy. Lancet 1996;347:1453–8.
38. Pearson JD. The endothelium: its role in scleroderma. Ann Rheum Dis 1991;50(Suppl 4):866–71.
39. Flavahan NA, Flavahan S, Liu Q, et al. Increased alpha2-adrenergic constriction of isolated arterioles in diffuse scleroderma. Arthritis Rheum 2000;43:1886–90.
40. Levin ER. Endothelins. N Engl J Med 1995;333:356–63.
41. Kahaleh MB. Endothelin, an endothelial-dependent vasoconstrictor in scleroderma. Enhanced production and profibrotic action. Arthritis Rheum 1991;34:978–83.
42. Yamane K, Miyauchi T, Suzuki N, et al. Significance of plasma endothelin-1 levels in patients with systemic sclerosis. J Rheumatol 1992;19:1566–71.

43. Vancheeswaran R, Magoulas T, Efrat G, et al. Circulating endothelin-1 levels in systemic sclerosis subsets–a marker of fibrosis or vascular dysfunction? J Rheumatol 1994;21:1838–44.
44. Kobayashi H, Nishimaki T, Kaise S, et al. Immunohistological study endothelin-1 and endothelin-A and B receptors in two patients with scleroderma renal crisis. Clin Rheumatol 1999;18:425–7.
45. Penn H, Quillinan N, Khan K, et al. Targeting the endothelin axis in scleroderma renal crisis: rationale and feasibility. QJM 2013;106(9):839–48.
46. Vancheeswaran R, Azam A, Black C, et al. Localization of endothelin-1 and its binding sites in scleroderma skin. J Rheumatol 1994;21:1268–76.
47. Rolla G, Colagrande P, Scappaticci E, et al. Exhaled nitric oxide in systemic sclerosis: relationships with lung involvement and pulmonary hypertension. J Rheumatol 2000;27:1693–8.
48. Andersen GN, Caidahl K, Kazzam E, et al. Correlation between increased nitric oxide production and markers of endothelial activation in systemic sclerosis: findings with the soluble adhesion molecules E-selectin, intercellular adhesion molecule 1, and vascular cell adhesion molecule 1. Arthritis Rheum 2000;43:1085–93.
49. Ibba-Manneschi L, Niissalo S, Milia AF, et al. Variations of neuronal nitric oxide synthase in systemic sclerosis skin. Arthritis Rheum 2006;54:202–13.
50. Carvalho D, Savage CO, Black CM, et al. IgG antiendothelial cell autoantibodies from scleroderma patients induce leukocyte adhesion to human vascular endothelial cells in vitro. Induction of adhesion molecule expression and involvement of endothelium-derived cytokines. J Clin Invest 1996;97:111–9.
51. Sgonc R, Gruschwitz MS, Boeck G, et al. Endothelial cell apoptosis in systemic sclerosis is induced by antibody-dependent cell-mediated cytotoxicity via CD95. Arthritis Rheum 2000;43:2550–62.
52. Ahmed SS, Tan FK, Arnett FC, et al. Induction of apoptosis and fibrillin 1 expression in human dermal endothelial cells by scleroderma sera containing anti-endothelial cell antibodies. Arthritis Rheum 2006;54:2250–62.
53. Sprott H, Müller-Ladner U, Distler O, et al. Detection of activated complement complex C5b-9 and complement receptor C5a in skin biopsies of patients with systemic sclerosis (scleroderma). J Rheumatol 2000;27:402–4.
54. Grote K, Flach I, Luchtefeld M, et al. Mechanical stretch enhances mRNA expression and proenzyme release of matrix metalloproteinase-2 (MMP-2) via NAD(P)H oxidase-derived reactive oxygen species. Circ Res 2003;92:e80–6.
55. Riccieri V, Spadaro A, Fuksa L, et al. Specific oxidative stress parameters differently correlate with nailfold capillaroscopy changes and organ involvement in systemic sclerosis. Clin Rheumatol 2008;27:225–30.
56. Kuwana M, Okazaki Y, Yasuoka H, et al. Defective vasculogenesis in systemic sclerosis. Lancet 2004;364:603–10.
57. Mulligan-Kehoe MJ, Drinane MC, Mollmark J, et al. Antiangiogenic plasma activity in patients with systemic sclerosis. Arthritis Rheum 2007;56:3448–58.
58. Springer TA. Adhesion receptors of the immune system. Nature 1990;346: 425–34.
59. Sato S. Abnormalities of adhesion molecules and chemokines in scleroderma. Curr Opin Rheumatol 1999;11:503–7.
60. Gruschwitz M, von den Driesch P, Kellner I, et al. Expression of adhesion proteins involved in cell-cell and cell-matrix interactions in the skin of patients with progressive systemic sclerosis. J Am Acad Dermatol 1992;27:169–77.
61. Carson CW, Beall LD, Hunder GG, et al. Serum ELAM-1 is increased in vasculitis, scleroderma, and systemic lupus erythematosus. J Rheumatol 1993;20:809–14.

62. Sfikakis PP, Tesar J, Baraf H, et al. Circulating intercellular adhesion molecule-1 in patients with systemic sclerosis. Clin Immunol Immunopathol 1993;68:88–92.
63. Stratton RJ, Coghlan JG, Pearson JD, et al. Different patterns of endothelial cell activation in renal and pulmonary vascular disease in scleroderma. QJM 1998;91:561–6.
64. Casciola-Rosen L, Wigley F, Rosen A. Scleroderma autoantigens are uniquely fragmented by metal-catalyzed oxidation reactions: implications for pathogenesis. J Exp Med 1997;185:71–9.
65. Chizzolini C, Raschi E, Rezzonico R, et al. Autoantibodies to fibroblasts induce a proadhesive and proinflammatory fibroblast phenotype in patients with systemic sclerosis. Arthritis Rheum 2002;46:1602–13.
66. Riemekasten G, Philippe A, Näther M, et al. Involvement of functional autoantibodies against vascular receptors in systemic sclerosis. Ann Rheum Dis 2011;70:530–6.
67. Baroni SS, Santillo M, Bevilacqua F, et al. Stimulatory autoantibodies to the PDGF receptor in systemic sclerosis. N Engl J Med 2006;354:2667–76.
68. Stummvoll GH, Aringer M, Grisar J, et al. Increased transendothelial migration of scleroderma lymphocytes. Ann Rheum Dis 2004;63:569–74.
69. Roumm AD, Whiteside TL, Medsger TA, et al. Lymphocytes in the skin of patients with progressive systemic sclerosis. Quantification, subtyping, and clinical correlations. Arthritis Rheum 1984;27:645–53.
70. Brent J, McMartin K, Phillips S, et al. Fomepizole for the treatment of ethylene glycol poisoning. Methylpyrazole for Toxic Alcohols Study Group. N Engl J Med 1999;340:832–8.
71. Murata M, Fujimoto M, Matsushita T, et al. Clinical association of serum interleukin-17 levels in systemic sclerosis: is systemic sclerosis a Th17 disease? J Dermatol Sci 2008;50:240–2.
72. Radstake TR, van Bon L, Broen J, et al. The pronounced Th17 profile in systemic sclerosis (SSc) together with intracellular expression of TGFbeta and IFNgamma distinguishes SSc phenotypes. PLoS One 2009;4:e5903.
73. Antiga E, Quaglino P, Bellandi S, et al. Regulatory T cells in the skin lesions and blood of patients with systemic sclerosis and morphoea. Br J Dermatol 2010;162:1056–63.
74. York MR. Novel insights on the role of the innate immune system in systemic sclerosis. Expert Rev Clin Immunol 2011;7:481–9.
75. Bhattacharyya S, Kelley K, Melichian DS, et al. Toll-like receptor 4 signaling augments transforming growth factor-β responses: a novel mechanism for maintaining and amplifying fibrosis in scleroderma. Am J Pathol 2013;182:192–205.
76. Abraham D, Lupoli S, McWhirter A, et al. Expression and function of surface antigens on scleroderma fibroblasts. Arthritis Rheum 1991;34:1164–72.
77. Higley H, Persichitte K, Chu S, et al. Immunocytochemical localization and serologic detection of transforming growth factor beta 1. Association with type I procollagen and inflammatory cell markers in diffuse and limited systemic sclerosis, morphea, and Raynaud's phenomenon. Arthritis Rheum 1994;37:278–88.
78. Corrin B, Butcher D, McAnulty BJ, et al. Immunohistochemical localization of transforming growth factor-beta 1 in the lungs of patients with systemic sclerosis, cryptogenic fibrosing alveolitis and other lung disorders. Histopathology 1994;24:145–50.

79. Dziadzio M, Smith RE, Abraham DJ, et al. Circulating levels of active transforming growth factor beta1 are reduced in diffuse cutaneous systemic sclerosis and correlate inversely with the modified Rodnan skin score. Rheumatology (Oxford) 2005;44:1518–24.

80. Kubo M, Ihn H, Yamane K, et al. Up-regulated expression of transforming growth factor beta receptors in dermal fibroblasts in skin sections from patients with localized scleroderma. Arthritis Rheum 2001;44:731–4.

81. McWhirter A, Colosetti P, Rubin K, et al. Collagen type I is not under autocrine control by transforming growth factor-beta 1 in normal and scleroderma fibroblasts. Lab. Invest 1994;71:885–94.

82. Yamakage A, Kikuchi K, Smith EA, et al. Selective upregulation of platelet-derived growth factor alpha receptors by transforming growth factor beta in scleroderma fibroblasts. J Exp Med 1992;175:1227–34.

83. Leask A, Holmes A, Abraham DJ. Connective tissue growth factor: a new and important player in the pathogenesis of fibrosis. Curr Rheumatol Rep 2002;4: 136–42.

84. Dziadzio M, Usinger W, Leask A, et al. N-terminal connective tissue growth factor is a marker of the fibrotic phenotype in scleroderma. QJM 2005;98:485–92.

85. Shi-wen X, Stanton LA, Kennedy L, et al. CCN2 is necessary for adhesive responses to transforming growth factor-beta1 in embryonic fibroblasts. J Biol Chem 2006;281:10715–26.

86. Andersen MB, Pingel J, Kjær M, et al. Interleukin-6: a growth factor stimulating collagen synthesis in human tendon. J Appl Physiol 2011;110:1549–54.

87. Sato S, Hasegawa M, Takehara K. Serum levels of interleukin-6 and interleukin-10 correlate with total skin thickness score in patients with systemic sclerosis. J Dermatol Sci 2001;27:140–6.

88. Salmon-Ehr V, Serpier H, Nawrocki B, et al. Expression of interleukin-4 in scleroderma skin specimens and scleroderma fibroblast cultures. Potential role in fibrosis. Arch Dermatol 1996;132:802–6.

89. Needleman BW, Wigley FM, Stair RW. Interleukin-1, interleukin-2, interleukin-4, interleukin-6, tumor necrosis factor α, and interferon-γ levels in sera from patients with scleroderma. Arthritis Rheum 1992;35:67–72.

90. Distler JH, Jüngel A, Caretto D, et al. Monocyte chemoattractant protein 1 released from glycosaminoglycans mediates its profibrotic effects in systemic sclerosis via the release of interleukin-4 from T cells. Arthritis Rheum 2006;54:214–25.

91. Aden N, Nuttall A, Shiwen X, et al. Epithelial cells promote fibroblast activation via IL-1alpha in systemic sclerosis. J Invest Dermatol 2010;130:2191–200.

92. Romagnani P, Maggi L, Mazzinghi B, et al. CXCR3-mediated opposite effects of CXCL10 and CXCL4 on TH1 or TH2 cytokine production. J Allergy Clin Immunol 2005;116:1372–9.

93. van Bon L, Affandi AJ, Broen J, et al. Proteome-wide analysis and CXCL4 as a biomarker in systemic sclerosis. N Engl J Med 2014;370:433–43.

94. Carulli MT, Ong VH, Ponticos M, et al. Chemokine receptor CCR2 expression by systemic sclerosis fibroblasts: evidence for autocrine regulation of myofibroblast differentiation. Arthritis Rheum 2005;52:3772–82.

95. Shi-Wen X, Denton CP, McWhirter A, et al. Scleroderma lung fibroblasts exhibit elevated and dysregulated type I collagen biosynthesis. Arthritis Rheum 1997; 40:1237–44.

96. Kähäri VM, Sandberg M, Kalimo H, et al. Identification of fibroblasts responsible for increased collagen production in localized scleroderma by in situ hybridization. J Invest Dermatol 1988;90:664–70.

97. Scharffetter K, Lankat-Buttgereit B, Krieg T. Localization of collagen mRNA in normal and scleroderma skin by in-situ hybridization. Eur J Clin Invest 1988; 18:9–17.

98. Denton CP, Khan K, Hoyles RK, et al. Inducible lineage-specific deletion of TbetaRII in fibroblasts defines a pivotal regulatory role during adult skin wound healing. J Invest Dermatol 2009;129:194–204.

99. Hoyles RK, Derrett-Smith EC, Khan K, et al. An essential role for resident fibroblasts in experimental lung fibrosis is defined by lineage-specific deletion of high-affinity type II transforming growth factor β receptor. Am J Respir Crit Care Med 2011;183:249–61.

100. LeRoy EC, Mercurio S, Sherer GK. Replication and phenotypic expression of control and scleroderma human fibroblasts: responses to growth factors. Proc Natl Acad Sci U S A 1982;79:1286–90.

101. Wang Y, Fan P-S, Kahaleh B. Association between enhanced type I collagen expression and epigenetic repression of the FLI1 gene in scleroderma fibroblasts. Arthritis Rheum 2006;54:2271–9.

102. Wallis DD, Tan FK, Kielty CM, et al. Abnormalities in fibrillin 1-containing microfibrils in dermal fibroblast cultures from patients with systemic sclerosis (scleroderma). Arthritis Rheum 2001;44:1855–64.

103. Lemaire R, Farina G, Kissin E, et al. Mutant fibrillin 1 from tight skin mice increases extracellular matrix incorporation of microfibril-associated glycoprotein 2 and type I collagen. Arthritis Rheum 2004;50:915–26.

New Classification Criteria for Systemic Sclerosis (Scleroderma)

Janet E. Pope, MD, MPH, FRCPC[a],*,
Sindhu R. Johnson, MD, PhD, FRCPC[b,c]

KEYWORDS

- Systemic sclerosis • Scleroderma • Classification criteria • Diagnosis • Validation
- Performance • Sensitivity • Specificity

KEY POINTS

- The American College of Rheumatology/European League Against Rheumatism classification criteria for systemic sclerosis (SSc) are more sensitive and specific than the previous 1980 American Rheumatism Association criteria for SSc.
- Classification criteria are not diagnostic criteria and were developed for clinical studies, but most patients diagnosed with SSc should meet classification criteria.
- There is no gold standard for SSc diagnosis and the criteria should only be applied if SSc diagnosis is suspected.

INTRODUCTION

Systemic sclerosis (SSc; also called scleroderma) refers to an autoimmune connective tissue disease with autoantibodies, vasculopathy, and fibrosis.[1] Most patients have sclerodactyly (thickened skin of the fingers) and may or may not have more extensive

Disclosure: The ACR/EULAR Classification Criteria for Systemic Sclerosis were funded by grants from the American College of Rheumatology (ACR) Classification and Response Criteria Subcommittee of the Committee on Quality Measures and the European League Against Rheumatism (EULAR). Dr J.E. Pope has no conflicts to declare. Dr S.R. Johnson is supported by a Canadian Institutes of Health Research Clinician Scientist Award and the Norton-Evans Fund for Scleroderma Research.
[a] Department of Medicine, St. Joseph's Health Care, University of Western Ontario, 268 Grosvenor Street, London, Ontario N6A 4V2, Canada; [b] Toronto Scleroderma Program, Division of Rheumatology, Department of Medicine, Toronto Western and Mount Sinai Hospitals, Ground Floor East Wing, 399 Bathurst Street, Toronto, Ontario M5T 2S8, Canada; [c] Institute of Health Policy, Management and Evaluation, University of Toronto, Ground Floor East Wing, 399 Bathurst Street, Toronto, Ontario M5T 2S8, Canada
* Corresponding author.
E-mail address: janet.pope@sjhc.london.on.ca

skin fibrosis. There are large differences in prevalence of internal organ involvement and other features, although nearly all have Raynaud phenomenon (RP), many have esophageal dysmotility, and 8% to 50% have pulmonary arterial hypertension (PAH), cardiac involvement, interstitial lung disease, inflammatory arthritis, and digital ulcers.[2] There is no laboratory test to diagnose SSc. With heterogeneous features and no diagnostic gold standard, it is important to classify patients with SSc along the disease spectrum as accurately as possible. Because SSc is rare, if a significant proportion of patients are not included in the classification then they will be missed when studying the disease.

Classification criteria are not diagnostic criteria. However, classification criteria should be similar to diagnostic criteria (with a large overlap of patients included in both criteria).[3] This article discusses the evolution of SSc classification criteria, strengths and weaknesses, and how to use the new American College of Rheumatology (ACR)/European League Against Rheumatism (EULAR) SSc classification criteria.

PREVIOUS SYSTEMIC SCLEROSIS CLASSIFICATION CRITERIA

Classification criteria have been published in SSc.[4–7] Classification criteria are used to include patients with a similar clinical entity for research studies,[3] but are used in a clinical setting to help to classify patients. The American Rheumatism Association (ARA) 1980 preliminary scleroderma (SSc) criteria were the most commonly cited criteria for SSc.[4,5,8] The 1980 preliminary scleroderma criteria were an important step in SSc classification.[4,5] There was 1 sufficient (major) criterion and 3 minor criteria. The major (sufficient) criterion was proximal cutaneous sclerosis/skin thickening (nonpitting) of the fingers that also extended proximal to the metacarpophalangeal joints (MCPs). If this criterion was not met, then at least 2 of 3 items had to be present: (1) sclerodactyly, (2) digital pitting scars of fingertips or loss of substance of the distal finger pad (digital tuft resorption), and (3) bibasilar pulmonary fibrosis.[4,5]

LIMITATIONS OF PREVIOUS CRITERIA

There are currently more patients with SSc who are at the mild end of the spectrum and in the limited cutaneous SSc subset (lcSSc) compared with patients in whom the 1980 criteria were tested, in whom a larger proportion of patients with diffuse cutaneous SSc (dcSSc) were identified; possibly because of the evolution of SSc over time, more recognition caused by available commercial autoantibodies, and/or earlier diagnosis. Many patients whom experts would now classify as SSc were not classified in the 1980 criteria. For example, a patient with sclerodactyly, telangiectasia, calcinosis, RP, proven PAH, and a positive anticentromere antibody test would not be classified as having SSc in the 1980 scheme. Patients with sclerodactyly, RP, anticentromere antibodies, dysphagia, dilated nail fold capillaries, and calcinosis would also not meet the previous criteria for SSc classification.

Often 20% of patients with lcSSc did not meet the criteria and were excluded from clinical studies.[1,9–11] This percentage means that 1 in 5 patients with lcSSc would not be classified with SSc even though they had a diagnosis of SSc.

OTHER PREVIOUSLY PROPOSED SYSTEMIC SCLEROSIS CLASSIFICATION CRITERIA

LeRoy and colleagues[12] proposed criteria that included clinical features, autoantibodies, and capillaroscopy. In 2001, LeRoy and Medsger[7] suggested revising the classification criteria to include early cases of SSc, using nail fold capillary changes and SSc-specific autoantibodies. The addition of nail fold capillary abnormalities and telangiectasia to the 1980 SSc criteria improves their sensitivity.[9,13] Adding RP to the 1980 criteria for SSc increased the number of patients classified with SSc.[6]

THE AMERICAN COLLEGE OF RHEUMATOLOGY/EUROPEAN LEAGUE AGAINST RHEUMATISM SYSTEMIC SCLEROSIS CLASSIFICATION CRITERIA

The ACR and the EULAR jointly funded the development of new SSc criteria, which was conducted in multiple phases. Candidate items for the classification criteria were identified through surveys of all potential items, followed by a Delphi process that reduced the 168 original features to 23 items.[14] Patients from international SSc cohorts were compared with control patients with diseases similar to SSc (mimickers) to test the discriminative ability of the items.[15] Next, SSc cases were purposively sampled from 2 European and 3 North American SSc centers to reflect the spectrum of probability that the subject could have SSc (ie, cases that had high probability, low probability, and in between). Data on the 23 candidate criteria for each of these cases were collected using a standardized form and provided to experts in a randomized order who ranked the cases from highest to lowest probability of having SSc.[16] A consensus meeting helped to define to whom the criteria should be applied (inclusion criteria: patients suspected of having SSc) and should not be applied (exclusion criteria: patients in whom a different diagnosis is far more likely and patients who have had skin fibrosis but without finger involvement), and which manifestations/items are sufficient to allow a patient to be classified as having SSc (sufficient criteria: sclerodactyly with continuous skin fibrosis proximal to the MCPs). Multicriteria decision analysis helped to determine the relative weighting of each of the items. Some items were deleted and some items were clustered (ie, the individual autoantibodies were grouped into an item about presence of SSc-related antibodies). Weights of items were rounded to whole numbers.[16–18] Cases were reranked with the scores of each item to determine a numerical threshold to exclude SSc cases that were less probable. There were cases for which all SSc experts thought the patients had SSc and others for which all agreed they did not have SSc, but there were also cases for which some experts thought the patient had SSc and others did not. Further cases were obtained and tested in this gray zone to identify a threshold that maintained specificity and sensitivity. A numerical range of the total score in this gray zone was tested in cases (patients with incident and prevalent SSc) and controls (SSc mimickers) that were prospectively collected at multiple sites and the data were divided randomly into derivation and validation cohorts. Low-frequency and statistically redundant items were removed. The resulting criteria were tested in the derivation sample of cases and controls and validated in the other sample. **Table 1** shows the ACR/EULAR SSc criteria. The sensitivity and specificity of the criteria were higher than for the 1980 criteria. In the validation sample, the 1980 criteria had a sensitivity of 75% and specificity of 73%, whereas the new criteria had greater than 90% sensitivity and specificity.

Using the American College of Rheumatology/European League Against Rheumatism Systemic Sclerosis Classification Criteria

The new ACR/EULAR SSc classification criteria are not to be applied if the patient has never had sclerodactyly but has fibrotic skin involvement elsewhere, thereby excluding eosinophilic fasciitis, generalized morphea, and other diseases that could be in the differential diagnosis of SSc. SSc mimickers were collected prospectively using cases and controls at multiple SSc sites, and from databases. Validation for the final ACR/EULAR SSc classification criteria was from the prospective cases and

Table 1
The ACR/EULAR criteria for the classification of SSc

Category	Subitems	Weight
Skin[a]	Skin thickening of the fingers of both hands extending proximal to the MCPs[b]	9
	Puffy fingers	2
	Whole finger, distal to MCP	4
Fingertip lesions[a]	Digital tip ulcers	2
	Pitting scars	3
Telangiectasia	—	2
Abnormal nail fold capillaries	—	2
PAH and/or interstitial lung disease	—	2
Raynaud's Phenomenon (RP)	—	3
Scleroderma-related antibodies (any of anticentromere, anti–topoisomerase-I [anti–Scl-70], anti–RNA polymerase-3)	—	3
—	Total score:	

These criteria are applicable to any patient considered for inclusion in an SSc study. Features can have been present at any time (ever).

Exclusion criteria: (1) these criteria are not applicable to patients having an SSc-like disorder better explaining their manifestations, such as nephrogenic sclerosing fibrosis, scleredema diabeticorum, scleromyxedema, erythromyalgia, porphyria, lichen sclerosis, graft-versus-host disease, and diabetic cheiroarthropathy; (2) patients with skin thickening that has never occurred on the fingers are also not classified as having SSc.

[a] Only the highest score from each category is used and the sum is totaled; a score of 9 or more classifies a patient as having SSc.

[b] Sufficient criterion: skin thickening of all fingers of both hands and extending proximal to the MCPs is sufficient for SSc classification (ie, it is scored as 9 and is sufficient for classification).

Adapted from van den Hoogen F, Khanna D, Fransen J, et al. 2013 classification criteria for systemic sclerosis: an American College of Rheumatology/European League Against Rheumatism collaborative initiative. Ann Rheum Dis 2013;72:1750; and van den Hoogen F, Khanna D, Fransen J, et al. 2013 classification criteria for systemic sclerosis: an American College of Rheumatology/European League Against Rheumatism collaborative initiative. Arthritis Rheum 2013;65:2741; with permission.

controls, including patients in whom the criteria would not be applied, so common sense and clinical judgment are needed to use the criteria. Expert opinion was used to reduce the number of potential items to be tested.

Methodological Advances

State-of-the-art methodology was used throughout the development of the 2013 SSc criteria establishing a comprehensive platform for classification criteria development in the modern era. Historical classification criteria in the rheumatic diseases have been threatened by a bias of circularity of reasoning in which investigators who developed classification criteria also contributed patient data in which the criteria were tested.[19] Through each phase of SSc criteria development, caution was taken to ensure that separate groups of investigators and centers were involved in data-driven and expert-based methods. This approach also resulted in broad geographic representation of experts and multiracial representation of patients throughout North

America and Europe. Candidate criteria were generated and reduced using advanced expert-based methods, including separate Delphi exercises in Europe and North America[14,20] and nominal group technique.[14] Multicriteria decision analysis facilitated further item reduction, weighting, and threshold identification.[16] Through these methods, years of expertise, knowledge, and experience were used to inform the criteria development in a manner that was least susceptible to bias. Bayesian methods were used to evaluate the ability of each proposed criterion to distinguish cases from controls, and the psychometric properties of face and construct validity of each criterion was evaluated.[15]

This methodological approach reflects increased collaboration between clinical experts and clinical epidemiologists; a balanced use of expert-based and data-driven methods, and implementation of bias reduction strategies and measurement science. This approach is being used to inform the development of classification criteria in other rheumatic diseases, including gout, myositis, and systemic lupus erythematosus (SLE).

Sensitivity and specificity were tested for the 2013 ACR/EULAR SSc classification criteria on serially collected patients from several outpatient clinics in Europe and North America. Approximately half the cases were early SSc so the performance of the new criteria in both established and early disease could be studied. The patients and controls (patients diagnosed with a disease that could mimic SSc) were from clinics that have expertise in SSc.

It was thought by experts in the 2013 criteria (using Delphi and other exercises) that some patients with mixed connective tissue disease (MCTD) could have SSc (overlaps were allowed) and some patients with current undifferentiated connective tissue could have several criteria for SSc (and perhaps be classified with SSc depending on the manifestations). A patient with MCTD with many features of SSc who scores 9 or more points in the 2013 ACR/EULAR SSc classification criteria would be classified as SSc and would presumably have a similar prognosis (when adjusting for the activity and severity of each SSc item) to other similar patients with SSc who do not have the other features of MCTD such as SLE, inflammatory myositis, or Sjögren syndrome features.

SSc disease may be a continuum (preclinical, mild, moderate, severe) with an arbitrary cutoff (above which the disease may be classified and below which the disease is not classified) and patients also may take time to meet criteria (undifferentiated connective tissue disease evolving into SSc). There were trade-offs between sensitivity and specificity at the 9 points needed for SSc classification and some experts classify patients with fewer criteria and occasionally do not classify a patient with SSc despite having the required 9 or more points.[16–18] There are trade-offs between having a simple useful classification scheme versus a more comprehensive one. Important SSc features were removed, such as scleroderma renal crisis (SRC) and calcinosis, because they were too rare (former) or did not add greater statistical value than the other included items (former and latter) or did not differentiate from other diseases in the differential diagnosis of SSc. Both the 1980 and the 2013 SSc classification systems allowed SSc sine (without) skin involvement (in the former meeting 2 of 3 minor criteria) and by scoring items other than skin involvement in the recent SSc classification.[4,5,17,18] The absolute criterion of skin involvement of the fingers and continuing proximal to the MCPs occurs in both schema. Examples of how to score cases are given later in this article.

STRENGTHS

The 2013 criteria incorporated the 3 main features of SSc: vasculopathy, fibrosis, and autoantibodies. RP was included as a feature because it does not distinguish from other patients with RP but it is so rare not to have RP in SSc that the item added statistical value to the criteria.[17,18]

In other cohorts, similar operational characteristics (sensitivity and specificity) have been reported.[21–24] These studies all reported that more patients in the lcSSc subset and with SSc sine scleroderma whom experts had classified as having SSc were classified with the ACR/EULAR criteria. The new criteria successfully capture more patients whom experts would classify as having SSc. The performance of the ACR/EULAR SSc criteria in an external cohort from Norway was similar to the criteria study validation cohort, as were the sensitivity and specificity of the 1980 criteria.[21] Sensitivity and specificity of any criteria also depend on the sample studied (ie, classification criteria are only applied when there is a high index of suspicion of SSc, and are not applied when a better explanation for the signs and symptoms is present). Examples of real patient cases are provided comparing the performance of the 1980 and ACR/EULAR criteria (**Table 2**). An ancillary table is also provided for practice scoring the SSc classification criteria (**Table 3**).

WEAKNESSES

As already noted, the classification criteria are not diagnostic criteria. For the 1980 and 2013 SSc classification criteria, patients are not classified with SSc if the only features are sclerodactyly (score of 4), gastroesophageal reflux disease (GERD) (score of 0), a dilated lower esophagus with retrosternal dysphagia (score of 0), and SRC (score of 0). Moreover, the RNA polymerase-3 antibody was not considered in the new criteria because it was not available in the local laboratory, reflecting the reality that many laboratories do not measure this antibody. Even if it had been included, it would only have added 3 more points to the case, for a total of 7, even though most experts are likely to consider such patients to have early and severe SSc. Over time, this patient could be classified if the scleroderma progressed from sclerodactyly alone to include skin involvement proximal to the MCPs (score of 9 instead of 4, which is a sufficient criterion to classify a patient with SSc). In this situation diagnosis of SSc and currently classifying the patient with SSc would be discordant but common sense would prevail and the patient appropriately treated with angiotensin II receptor antagonist with the addition of other antihypertensives as needed to achieve normotension as quickly as possible. If a study were designed to treat scleroderma renal crisis, perhaps the inclusion criterion would be broader than demanding a patient meet the new ACR EULAR SSc classification because SRC often occurs as the initial presentation of SSc, perhaps associated with puffy fingers and recent onset of RP.

Another weakness is that criteria may not include borderline cases (eg, a large proportion of SSc experts not classifying the patient as having SSc), as well as early patients.

Also, items in the classification could have occurred previously and then no longer be present, such as dilated capillaries and even sclerodactyly. If there is certainty that an item has ever been present, then it is scored. A patient with a decade of SSc disease may have nail fold capillary dropout so none are currently seen with low-level magnification and the patient may no longer have RP with pallor.

Item definitions are open to interpretation. **Fig. 1** shows an example of when not to apply the SSc criteria, and items such as skin thickening, fingertip lesions, telangiectasia, abnormal nail fold capillaries, and RP are show in **Figs. 2–6**. Telangiectasia in SSc may be dotlike or mattlike (the latter often occurs with long disease durations; see **Fig. 4**). Telangiectasia in a scleroderma-like pattern seems to be circular reasoning as the patterns increase the likelihood of the patient having scleroderma and the definition for telangiectasia has scleroderma in it.

Table 2
A comparison of 1980 and 2013 ACR/EULAR SSc classification criteria

Features	Meeting 1980 Preliminary SSc Criteria	Meeting 2013 ACR/EULAR SSc Classification Criteria[a]
Sclerodactyly and skin thickening proximal to the MCPs	Yes	Yes (score is 9)
Sclerodactyly of fingers, digital pits	Yes	Not necessarily; depends on what other features may be present If whole finger score is 4, if only distal finger, score is 0 Digital pits score is 3 Total score could be 7
Sclerodactyly, interstitial lung disease with bilateral pulmonary fibrosis	Yes	Not necessarily; depends on what other features may be present If whole finger score is 4, if only distal finger, score is 0 Interstitial lung disease score is 2 Total could be 6
Sclerodactyly of entire fingers, RP, PAH, positive anticentromere antibody	No (only 1 minor criterion is met)	Yes Sclerodactyly, 4 RP, 3 PAH, 2 Positive anticentromere antibody, 3 Total score, 12
Sclerodactyly, RP, positive anticentromere antibody, dysphagia, dilated nail fold capillaries, calcinosis	No (only 1 minor criterion is met)	Sclerodactyly, 4 RP, 3 Positive anticentromere antibody, 3 Dysphagia, 0 Abnormal Nail fold capillaries, 2 Calcinosis, 0 Total score, 12
Sclerodactyly, ILD, RP, positive topoisomerase-1 antibody	Yes (2 minor criteria)	Yes Sclerodactyly, 4 ILD, 2 RP, 3 Positive topoisomerase-1 antibody, 3 Total score, 12
Sclerodactyly whole fingers, RP, SRC, positive RNA polymerase-3 antibody	No (1 minor criterion)	Yes Sclerodactyly, 4 RP, 3 SRC, 0 Positive RNA polymerase-3, 3 Total score, 10

(continued on next page)

Table 2 (continued)		
Features	**Meeting 1980 Preliminary SSc Criteria**	**Meeting 2013 ACR/EULAR SSc Classification Criteria[a]**
Sclerodactyly whole fingers, RP, SRC, RNA polymerase-3 antibody not available	No (1 minor criterion)	No Sclerodactyly, 4 RP, 3 SRC, 0 Total score, 7
SLE with malar rash, photosensitivity, low WBC, +ANA, +anticentromere Ab fingertip ulcers, puffy fingers RP, telangiectasia, calcinosis, needing repeat esophageal dilations	No (perhaps no minor criteria are met because puffy fingers may not be considered sclerodactyly and there are fingertip ulcers but no pitting scars)	Yes + anticentromere Ab, 3 Fingertip ulcers, 2 Puffy fingers, 2 RP, 3 Telangiectasia, 2 Calcinosis, 0 Needing repeat esophageal dilations, 0 Total score, 12

Abbreviations: +, positive; Ab, antibody; ANA, antinuclear antibody; ILD, interstitial lung disease; PAH, pulmonary arterial hypertension; WBC, white blood cell count.

[a] A score of 9 or more is necessary to classify SSc.

The 2013 criteria included patients from North America and Europe. Patients with SSc from other countries have different proportions of various items such as presence of autoantibodies. For instance, the distributions of anticentromere and topoisomerase antibodies vary between the United States and China.[25] This finding is also likely true for other regions where the distribution between lcSSc and dcSSc and autoantibodies may be different from North America and Europe.[26-31]

Table 3 Comparison of the 1980 and ACR/EULAR SSc classification criteria		
Cases	**Meeting SSc 1980 Classification Criteria**	**Meeting ACR/EULAR SSc Classification Criteria**
Sclerodactyly, calcinosis, RP, positive anticentromere, PAH	No	Yes
Sclerodactyly, tendon friction rubs, dilated esophagus retrosternally on chest radiograph, dysphagia, positive RNA polymerase-3, SRC	No	Yes
Sclerodactyly of whole fingers, RP, anticentromere, dysphagia, dilated nail fold capillaries, calcinosis	No	Yes
Diffuse SSc: sclerodactyly and proximal skin involvement including hands, arms, trunk, face	Yes	Yes
Modified Rodnan skin score of 20 and no finger involvement ever, no RP, and negative ANA (generalized morphea)	No	No

Abbreviations: PAH, pulmonary arterial hypertension; RP, raynaud's phenomenon; SSc, systemic clerosis.

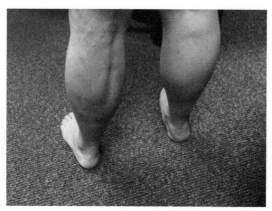

Fig. 1. When not to apply SSc criteria: Linear Scleroderma.

In the development of these criteria, clinical databases from several scleroderma centers were acquired and combined. Some databases did not collect all variables of interest and definitions for items may have been different or not standardized. Random samples of available databases were combined for item reduction and to determine face validity of potential criteria.[14,15]

As mentioned earlier, RNA polymerase-3 antibody is not widely available, which limits application of the scleroderma-specific autoantibodies. More antibodies may be used in the future and the new criteria do not limit their application, but the sensitivity and specificity could change if new antibodies are added to this category.

Some experts may consider patients with early signs and symptoms of connective tissue disease and some features of SSc (eg, anticentromere antibody, RP, and abnormal nail fold capillaries) as having probable SSc, pre-SSc, or early SSc. The new ACR/EULAR criteria do not classify these patients as having SSc when they have only these features because they score 3 points for RP, 2 for abnormal nail fold capillaries, and 3 for a SSc-related autoantibody for a total score of 8, whereas 9 is the threshold to classify SSc. The idea of very early SSc or pre-SSc has been discussed in a recent review.[32] When developing the new criteria, there were trade-offs between sensitivity and specificity. For instance, criteria that are too sensitive misclassify more patients who do not have this rare disease, and, if too specific, they do not include patients whom many experts would classify as SSc. When SSc experts classified cases as SSc or not (from patients with a spectrum of probability of having SSc), the cutoff to classify patients with SSc was when at least 70% of experts considered the patient to have SSc. We did not want an overly sensitive criteria set that would misclassify someone with SSc who did not have the disease, because the diagnosis of SSc has repercussions to an individual with respect to screening, prognosis, and ability to obtain life/health insurance, and it also carries an emotional burden. In a rare disease, overclassifying patients (false-positives) potentially leads to the classification of large numbers of people who do not have SSc, such as those with low-grade connective tissue diseases with different prognoses than SSc.

Definitions of Items in the American College of Rheumatology/European League Against Rheumatism Systemic Sclerosis Classification

An item can ever have been present (so not necessarily currently) and, when a satisfactory definition was not available in the literature, a consensus was achieved. Skin

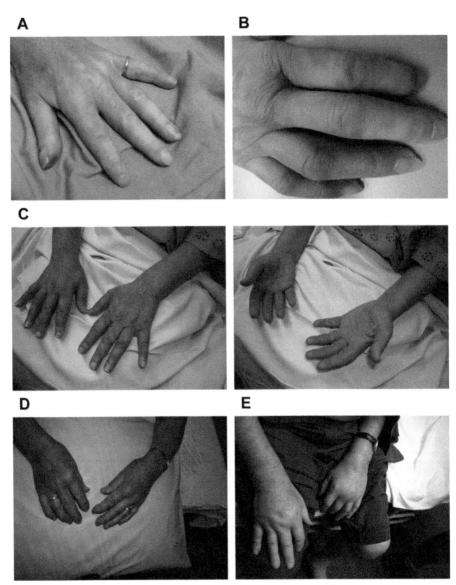

Fig. 2. Skin thickening. (*A*) Sufficient criterion: skin thickening of fingers proximal to MCPs. (*B*) Sclerodactyly not proximal to MCPs. (*C*) Puffy fingers. (*C Part 2*) Puffy fingers from palmar view; note telangiectasia. (*D*) Puffy fingers in a patient with SSc. (*E*) Not puffy fingers; swelling is caused by tenosynovitis.

thickening was considered hardening or thickening of the skin not of other causes. Likewise, puffy fingers were not caused by edema or inflammatory dactylitis. The definition or measurement of some criterion items was not usually given, such as method of antibody testing or cutoff for a positive result, in order to have the criterion work in the usual clinical setting. Similarly how abnormal nail fold capillary patterns were identified was not specified (ie, with no magnification or with use of magnification such as magnified polarizing light instruments, otoscopes, ophthalmoscopes, microscopes,

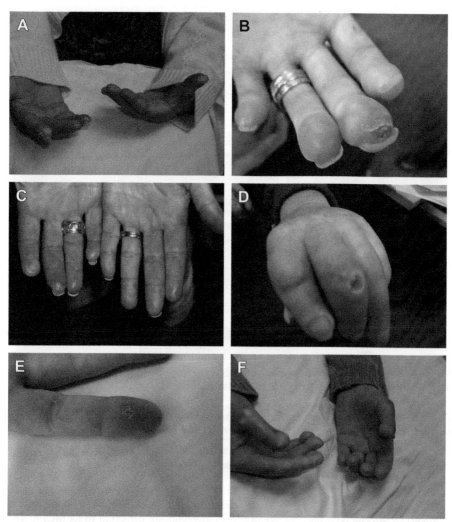

Fig. 3. Fingertip lesions. (*A*) Digital tip ulcers R2, R4, and L1 digits. (*B*) Healing digital ulcer. (*C*) Pitting scars on second and third right fingers. (*D*) Ulcer from SSc but not a digital tip ulcer. (*E*) This is not a digital tip ulcer. (*F*) Not part of ACR/EULAR SSc criteria, but this was part of 1980 SSc criteria for loss of substance of the distal finger pads.

and capillaroscopy, or by other methods). Interstitial lung disease could be diagnosed in several ways (eg, chest radiograph, high-resolution computed tomography [CT] scan, restrictive pattern on pulmonary function tests), whereas PAH is to be diagnosed by current criteria using right heart catheterization or by other standardized means if criteria evolve over time. Telangiectasia could be either round and well demarcated in classic areas such as the hands and lips or mattlike, and other causes or types of telangiectasia would be excluded from this definition (such as those found in liver disease or acne rosacea). Fingertip ulcers or pits would exclude other causes (such as trauma). RP could be self-reported or witnessed with at least 2 color phases (usually pallor but could be rubor and/or cyanosis).

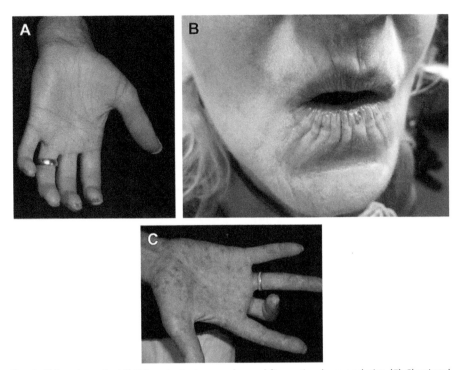

Fig. 4. Telangiectasia. (*A*) Telangiectasia on palm and fingertip ulcers and pits. (*B*) Classic telangiectasia on mouth. (*C*) Mattlike telangiectasia.

Cases Examples of Scoring for the American College of Rheumatology/European League Against Rheumatism Systemic Sclerosis Classification Criteria

There is an Internet calculator available for scoring the ACR/EULAR SSc classification criteria at rheuminfo.com/physician-tools/ssc-calculator on the RheumInfo Web site.

Case 1

The patient has had RP for 5 months and scleroderma of the skin with all fingers involved (sclerodactyly) and contiguous skin involvement proximal to all MCPs. The patient also has bilateral basilar pulmonary fibrosis of the bases of the lungs on chest

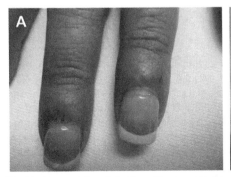
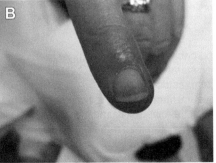

Fig. 5. Abnormal nail fold capillaries. (*A*) Abnormal nail fold capillaries (also seen on the cuticle of the third finger). (*B*) Abnormal nail fold capillaries.

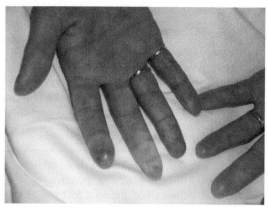

Fig. 6. Raynaud's Phenomenon (RP).

radiograph and confirmed with high-resolution CT scan of the lungs and with a moderate restrictive lung pattern on pulmonary function tests. This patient has a sufficient criterion (sclerodactyly with skin thickening also proximal to the MCPs). This scores criterion 9 and, if desired, the other features can be added, such as RP (scores 3) and interstitial lung disease (ILD) (scores 2). The total score is 14. This patient could be in either the diffuse (dcSSc) or limited (lcSSc) subset, and that depends on the extent of skin involvement (ie, whether the scleroderma skin changes were proximal to the elbows and/or knees or truncal), but either subset could have involvement of the face and neck (scores 12). There is no need to add the items if the sufficient criterion is met (sclerodactyly with contiguous skin involvement proximal to the MCPs).

Case 2
A patient has RP (scores 3), sclerodactyly (scores 4), telangiectasia (scores 2), calcinosis (scores 0), need for repeated esophageal dilations (scores 0), fingertip ulcers (scores 2), and a positive anticentromere antibody (scores 3) (scoring 14). Another patient has diffuse cutaneous skin involvement with sclerodactyly proximal to the MCPs (scores 9), a very high modified Rodnan skin score of 30, tendon friction rubs (scores 0), PAH (scores 2), RP (scores 3), antinuclear antibody (ANA) in a nucleolar pattern (scores 0), and the ENA is negative but RNA polymerase-3 is unavailable (scores 0). This patient also has a score of 14 but has a worse prognosis because PAH is a lethal complication and the rapid progression of skin involvement with tendon friction rubs is associated with a higher chance of other organ involvement. Equal scores do not translate into the same prognosis. A higher score does not mean necessarily a worse prognosis or disease burden.

Case 3
A patient with a diagnosis of SSc has ILD (scores 2), proven PAH (not counted as an extra 2 points because this category is already scored for ILD), digital pits (scores 3), a current fingertip ulcer (scores 2, but not counted because the patient has digital pits), a positive ANA test in a centromere pattern (scores 3), and anticentromere antibody was positive when performed previously (scores 3, but not scored because anticentromere is already scored). Sclerodactyly of the entire fingers just distal to the MCPs (scores 4) is present and fingers are puffy (scores 2, but not counted because sclerodactyly is scored). This patient scores a total of 12. Count only the highest score in each category.

Case 4: systemic sclerosis overlapping with Sjögren's syndrome

A 64-year-old woman has sicca with both dry eyes and dry mouth. She has a positive salivary gland biopsy with lymphocytic infiltration and a positive Schirmer test. She has been diagnosed with Sjögren's syndrome. She also has had RP for years (scores 3); puffy fingers (scores 2); a positive anticentromere antibody test (scores 3); calcinosis (scores 0); retrosternal esophageal dysphagia (scores 0); and many dot telangiectasias of the hands, lips, and inside her mouth (scores 2). She meets classification criteria for SSc with a score of 10. A patient can have another diagnosis and still be classified with SSc.

Case 5: systemic sclerosis sine scleroderma

A patient has never had skin involvement, but has classic telangiectasia, PAH shown by right heart catheterization, RP for years, a positive ANA test with positive topoisomerase-1 antibody. This person is thought to have SSc sine scleroderma and scores telangiectasia (2), PAH (2), RP (3), positive ANA (0 because it is not in a centromere pattern), and a scleroderma-related autoantibody test (3), totaling 10. This is more than the threshold of 9. The patient may also have GERD, dysphagia that is retrosternal, calcinosis, and gastric antral vascular ectasia, all of which increase the likelihood of diagnosing SSc but do not increase the item score. The score of 9 or more classifies this patient with SSc. There may never have been skin involvement but the patient could have SSc.

Case 6

A 54-year-old man has eosinophilia and tight, woody skin of the arms and legs. There is no RP and there has never been sclerodactyly. There is no GERD, no dilated nail fold capillaries, and no other items are present in the SSc classification criteria. The ACR/EULAR SSc classification criteria are not applied because eosinophilic fasciitis is suspected. The same logic would apply if a person has been diagnosed with generalized morphea without any finger involvement ever and no features of SSc (eg, negative ANA and negative ENA tests, no RP, no GERD, no calcinosis, no pits or digital ulcers). Do not apply the criteria if a better explanation is considered.

FUTURE CONSIDERATIONS/SUMMARY

Several publications are likely to show that the ACR/EULAR criteria have very good specificity and sensitivity but that they are not perfect. SSc subset criteria are an important next step because subsets may correlate with prognosis.[33] Subsets could be divided by the extent of skin involvement (anatomic location, maximum ever), autoantibodies, or by organ involvement. Previous criteria for the lcSSc and dcSSc subsets are used in many clinics.[12] There are limitations to these criteria even though they correlate with some organ involvement and mortality; autoantibodies may also help to predict prognosis and are not in the current 2 subsets. Early patients may be considered to have lcSSc but, as skin evolves, the condition can become dcSSc and likewise, as skin regresses, patients with dcSSc can convert to lcSSc. Subtypes could also include overlaps, sine skin involvement, and very early patients.[34,35]

Phenotypes could be divided by genotypes, protein or gene expression data, or other molecular differences, but these techniques are not ready for clinical use.[36] In the future, the 2013 criteria are likely to be outdated as understanding of SSc evolves.

At present the ACR/EULAR SSc classification has superior sensitivity and specificity compared with the 1980 criteria, and especially performs better in the lcSSc subset, which lacks pulmonary fibrosis or digital pitting scars.

REFERENCES

1. Wollheim FA. Classification of systemic sclerosis: visions and reality. Rheumatology (Oxford) 2005;44:1212–6.
2. Muangchan C, Canadian Scleroderma Research Group, Baron M, et al. The 15% rule in scleroderma: the frequency of severe organ complications in systemic sclerosis. A systematic review. J Rheumatol 2013;40(9):1545–56.
3. Singh JA, Solomon DH, Dougados M, et al. Development of classification and response criteria for rheumatic diseases. Arthritis Rheum 2006;55:348–52.
4. Masi AT, Rodnan G, Medsger T, et al. Preliminary criteria for the classification of systemic sclerosis (scleroderma). Subcommittee for scleroderma criteria of the American Rheumatism Association. Diagnostic and Therapeutic Criteria Committee. Arthritis Rheum 1980;23(5):581–90.
5. Preliminary criteria for the classification of systemic sclerosis (scleroderma). Bull Rheum Dis 1981;31:1–6.
6. Nadashkevich O, Davis P, Fritzler MJ. A proposal of criteria for the classification of systemic sclerosis. Med Sci Monit 2004;10(11):CR615–21.
7. LeRoy EC, Medsger TA Jr. Criteria for the classification of early systemic sclerosis. J Rheumatol 2001;28(7):1573–6.
8. Johnson SR, Goek ON, Singh-Grewal D, et al. Classification criteria in rheumatic diseases. A review of methodologic properties. Arthritis Rheum 2007;57(7):1119–33.
9. Lonzetti LS, Joyal F, Raynauld JP, et al. Updating the American College of Rheumatology preliminary classification criteria for systemic sclerosis: addition of severe nailfold capillaroscopy abnormalities markedly increases the sensitivity for limited scleroderma. Arthritis Rheum 2001;44(3):735–6.
10. Hachulla E, Launay D. Diagnosis and classification of systemic sclerosis. Clin Rev Allergy Immunol 2011;40(2):78–83.
11. Walker JG, Pope J, Baron M, et al. The development of systemic sclerosis classification criteria. Clin Rheumatol 2007;26(9):1401–9.
12. LeRoy EC, Black C, Fleischmajer R, et al. Scleroderma (systemic sclerosis): classification, subsets and pathogenesis. J Rheumatol 1988;15(2):202–5.
13. Hudson M, Taillefer S, Steele R, et al. Improving the sensitivity of the American College of Rheumatology classification criteria for systemic sclerosis. Clin Exp Rheumatol 2007;25(5):754–7.
14. Fransen J, Johnson SR, van den Hoogen F, et al. Items for developing revised classification criteria in systemic sclerosis: results of a consensus exercise. Arthritis Care Res 2012;64:351–7.
15. Johnson SR, Fransen J, Khanna D, et al. Validation of potential classification criteria for systemic sclerosis. Arthritis Care Res 2012;64(3):358–67.
16. Johnson SR, Naden RP, Fransen J, et al. Scleroderma classification criteria: developing methods for multi-criteria decision analysis using 1000 minds. J Clin Epidemiol 2014;67(6):706–14.
17. van den Hoogen F, Khanna D, Fransen J, et al. 2013 classification criteria for systemic sclerosis: an American college of Rheumatology/European League Against Rheumatism collaborative initiative. Ann Rheum Dis 2013;72:1747–55.
18. van den Hoogen F, Khanna D, Fransen J, et al. 2013 classification criteria for systemic sclerosis: an American College Of Rheumatology/European League Against Rheumatism collaborative initiative. Arthritis Rheum 2013;65:2737–47.
19. Felson DT, Anderson JJ. Methodologic and statistical approaches to criteria development in rheumatic diseases. Baillieres Clin Rheumatol 1995;9:253–66.

20. Coulter C, Baron M, Pope JE. A Delphi exercise and cluster analysis to aid in the development of potential classification criteria for systemic sclerosis using SSc experts and databases. Clin Exp Rheumatol 2013;31(2 Suppl 76):24–30.

21. Hoffmann-Vold A-M, Gunnarsson R, Garen T, et al. Performance of the 2013 ACR/EULAR classification criteria for systemic sclerosis (SSc) in large, well defined cohorts of SSc and mixed connective tissue disease. J Rheumatol 2015;42:60–3.

22. Alhajeri H, Hudson M, Fritzler M, et al, Canadian Scleroderma Research Group (CSRG). Evaluation of the new ACR/EULAR criteria for the classification of systemic sclerosis in the Canadian Scleroderma Research Group cohort. J Rheumatol 2014;41:1530–1.

23. Yaqub A, Chung L, Fiorentino D, et al. Validation of the ICD-CM-9 code for systemic sclerosis using updated ACR/EULAR classification criteria. Arthritis Rheum 2013;65:S772–3.

24. Andréasson K, Saxne T, Bergknut C, et al. Prevalence and incidence of systemic sclerosis in southern Sweden: population-based data with case ascertainment using the 1980 ARA criteria and the proposed ACR-EULAR classification criteria. Ann Rheum Dis 2014;73(10):1788–92.

25. Wang J, Assassi S, Guo G, et al. Clinical and serological features of systemic sclerosis in a Chinese cohort. Clin Rheumatol 2013;32(5):617–21.

26. Hashimoto A, Endo H, Kondo H, Hirohata S. Clinical features of 405 Japanese patients with systemic sclerosis. Mod Rheumatol 2012;22(2):272–9.

27. Graf SW, Hakendorf P, Lester S, et al. South Australian Scleroderma Register: autoantibodies as predictive biomarkers of phenotype and outcome. Int J Rheum Dis 2012;15(1):102–9.

28. Müller Cde S, Paiva Edos S, Azevedo VF, et al. Autoantibody profile and clinical correlation in a group of patients with systemic sclerosis in southern Brazil. Rev Bras Reumatol 2011;51(4):314–8, 323–4.

29. Admou B, Arji N, Seghrouchni F, et al. Low prevalence of anti-centromere antibodies in scleroderma in Morocco (about 272 cases). Ann Biol Clin (Paris) 2007;65(3):291–7.

30. Pradhan V, Rajadhyaksha A, Nadkar M, et al. Clinical and autoimmune profile of scleroderma patients from Western India. Int J Rheumatol 2014;2014:983781.

31. Gottschalk P, Vásquez R, López PD, et al. Scleroderma in the Caribbean: characteristics in a Dominican case series. Rheumatol Clin 2014;10(6):373–9.

32. Valentini G, Marcoccia A, Cuomo G, et al. The concept of early systemic sclerosis following 2013 ACR\EULAR criteria for the classification of systemic sclerosis. Curr Rheumatol Rev 2014;10(1):38–44.

33. Johnson SR, Feldman BM, Hawker GA. Classification criteria for scleroderma subsets. J Rheumatol 2007;34:1855–63.

34. Matucci-Cerinic M, Bellando-Randone S, Lepri G, et al. Very early versus early disease: the evolving definition of the 'many faces' of systemic sclerosis. Ann Rheum Dis 2013;72(3):319–21.

35. Pope JE. SSc classification: a rose by any other name would smell as sweet? J Rheumatol 2015;42(1):11–3.

36. Varga J, Hinchcliff M. Connective tissue diseases: systemic sclerosis: beyond limited and diffuse subsets? Nat Rev Rheumatol 2014;10(4):200–2.

Management of Systemic Sclerosis-Related Skin Disease

A Review of Existing and Experimental Therapeutic Approaches

Elizabeth R. Volkmann, MD, MS*, Daniel E. Furst, MD

KEYWORDS

- Diffuse cutaneous systemic sclerosis (DcSSc)
- Limited cutaneous systemic sclerosis (LcSSc) • Modified Rodnan skin score (mRSS)
- Digital ulcers (DU) • Raynaud's phenomenon (RP) • Methotrexate (MTX)
- Cyclophosphamide (CYC) • Hematopoietic stem cell transplantation (HSCT)

KEY POINTS

- The hallmark of systemic sclerosis (SSc) is cutaneous sclerosis, affecting nearly all patients with this rare and debilitating autoimmune disorder.
- Patients with SSc are classified based on the distribution of cutaneous involvement (ie, limited vs diffuse), and this distinction has important clinical implications.
- Existing treatment options for diffuse cutaneous SSc-cutaneous sclerosis include methotrexate, cyclophosphamide, and hematopoietic stem cell transplantation. Less evidence exists for treatment of limited cutaneous LcSSc-cutaneous sclerosis.
- All SSc patients experience Raynaud's phenomenon. After general preventative measures are taken, calcium channel blockers, prostacyclin analogs, and phosphodiesterase type 5 inhibitors are often used.
- A paucity of evidence is available for the management of digital ulcers, cutaneous telangiectasias, calcinosis, and pigment changes.

Disclosure Statement: E.R. Volkmann has no disclosures. D.E. Furst reports the following disclosures: D.E. Furst is a consultant for AbbVie, Actelion, Amgen, BMS, Cytori, Janssen, Gilead, GSK, NIH, Novartis, Pfizer, Roche/Genentech, UCB.
Division of Rheumatology, Department of Medicine, David Geffen School of Medicine, University of California, Los Angeles, 1000 Veteran Avenue, Suite 32-59, Los Angeles, CA 90095, USA
* Corresponding author.
E-mail address: Evolkmann@mednet.ucla.edu

INTRODUCTION

Virtually all patients with systemic sclerosis (SSc) experience cutaneous sclerosis and Raynaud's phenomenon (RP), although substantial variability in the presentation and severity of these cutaneous manifestations exist. Moreover, many patients with SSc exhibit varying degrees of additional and often disabling cutaneous manifestations, such as digital ulcers (DU), cutaneous telangiectasias, calcinosis, and pigment changes. The inherent heterogeneity in these cutaneous manifestations complicates strategies for improving patient care, as well as clinical trial design.[1,2] This review examines skin changes in SSc and how to manage them.

SYMPTOMS
Skin Sclerosis

The hallmark of SSc is skin thickening and hardening.[1] Symptoms usually first develop in the fingers and hands. Many patients experience nonpitting edema, erythema, and pruritus before the development of skin induration. Subsequently, the skin becomes firm and taut, adhering to deeper structures and limiting movement (**Fig. 1**). The presence of skin thickening of the fingers extending proximally to the metacarpophalangeal joints is characteristic of SSc and alone is sufficient to classify a patient as having SSc.[2]

As the disease progresses, the epidermis of the skin atrophies, leading to impaired hair growth and decreased sweating (ie, anhydrosis). Normal skin creases vanish, and the skin can seem to be shiny and undergo pigmentary changes. The combination of atrophy and sclerosis overflexed joints combined with a vasculopathy and dermal inflammation can cause ulceration and a reactive hyperkeratosis. The majority of patients have facial skin sclerosis, producing characteristic changes around the mouth, including increased furrowing of the skin around the lips, recession of the lips, and decreased oral aperture.

The distribution of cutaneous involvement has been classically based on the maximum extent of skin involvement.[1] In patients with diffuse cutaneous SSc (DcSSc), skin thickening occurs proximally to the elbows or knees (as well as finger/hand involvement), and often involves the trunk, whereas in patients with limited cutaneous SSc (LcSSc), skin thickening is confined to the distal extremities, or may only affect the fingers (ie, sclerodactyly; **Fig. 2**). Facial involvement is common and contributes to

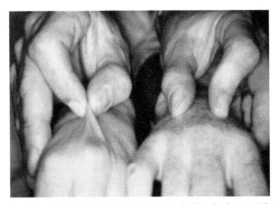

Fig. 1. Skin thickening. The left dorsal hand has normal skin thickness. The right dorsal hand has increased skin thickness. (*Courtesy of* P. Clements, MD.)

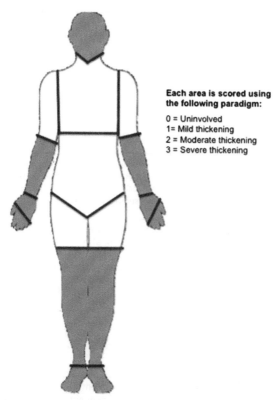

Each area is scored using
the following paradigm:

0 = Uninvolved
1 = Mild thickening
2 = Moderate thickening
3 = Severe thickening

Fig. 2. Schematic for the Modified Rodnan Skin Score (mRSS). Total mRSS equals the sum of the following individual areas: face, chest, abdomen, right upper arm, left upper arm, right forearm, left forearm, right hand, left hand, right fingers, left fingers, right thigh, left thigh, right leg, left leg, right foot, and left foot. Purple skin denotes limited skin involvement and white skin denotes diffuse skin involvement.

neither classification nor prognosis. The distinction between limited and diffuse cutaneous involvement has prognostic implications for patients.[3] In fewer than 5% of patients, there is no skin thickening and these patients are classified as SSc sine skin sclerosis/scleroderma.

Nonsclerotic Skin Manifestations

The key nonsclerotic features of SSc are summarized in **Table 1**.

DIAGNOSIS
Physical Examination

The diagnosis of SSc is usually made on clinical grounds, with supporting laboratory studies.[2] Skin thickening is easily detectable on physical examination and can be reasonably quantified using the validated modified Rodnan skin score (mRSS).[8] Skin thickness at 17 anatomic sites is assessed by palpation and rated on a scale of 0 (normal), 1 (mild), 2 (moderate), or 3 (severe) skin thickening (see **Fig. 2**). The total skin score is the sum of the individual skin assessments and the within-patient variability in scoring is approximately 5 units.[9] The minimal, clinically discernible difference is 4 to 5.1.[10] Ultrasound approaches are being tested, but are not yet validated.[11]

Table 1
Nonsclerotic skin manifestations of systemic sclerosis

Symptom	Overall Prevalence in SSc	Distribution	Onset of Timing
Raynaud's phenomenon	>95% overall	Hands, usually asymmetric initially (**Fig. 3**)	LcSSc: Can precede skin sclerosis by several years DcSSc: Usually precedes onset of skin sclerosis by <1 y
Ischemic ulceration	LcSSc: ~38% DcSSc: ~50%	Digital tips most common (**Fig. 4**); Also occurs on extensor surfaces of joints	LcSSc or DcSSc: Finger tip ulcers associated with vasculopathy so may occur early or late
Calcinosis	LcSSc: ~40% DcSSc: ~24%	Fingers most common (**Fig. 5**); also commonly occurs around trauma sites, such as elbows, knees, buttocks, feet	LcSSc: Usually the product of damaged tissue in the presence of vasculopathy, so often late, but can occur early DcSSc: Typically late-stage disease
Telangiectasia	LcSSc: ~85% DcSSc: ~84%	Fingers, lips, and face most common	LcSSc and DcSSc: Late-stage disease more common, but can occur early
Pigment changes	Majority of both LcSSc and DcSSc (more easily seen in Hispanics and African Americans)	Hyperpigmentation: Face, lower abdomen and thighs most common Acanthosis nigricans-like changes: Flexure surfaces Vitiligo-like loss of pigment Perifollicular distribution common (salt and pepper)	LcSSc: Typically late-stage disease DcSSc: Typically late-stage disease
Cutaneous vasculitis with ulceration	More common in LcSSc	Palpable purpura: Lower extremities Deep ulcerations: Lower extremities	LcSSc and DcSSc: Typically late stage disease

Abbreviations: DcSSc, diffuse cutaneous systemic sclerosis; LcSSc, limited cutaneous systemic sclerosis.
Data from Refs.[4–7]

Nonsclerotic skin manifestations (see **Table 1**), such as digital tip ulcers, RP, and telangiectasias, can support a diagnosis of SSc, as documented by the 2013 European League Against Rheumatism (EULAR)/American College of Rheumatology (ACR) SSc criteria.[2] In addition, enlarged capillaries and/or capillary dropout with or without pericapillary hemorrhages may be appreciated at the nailfold and may predict future organ involvement, although there remains much to be done in this area.[12]

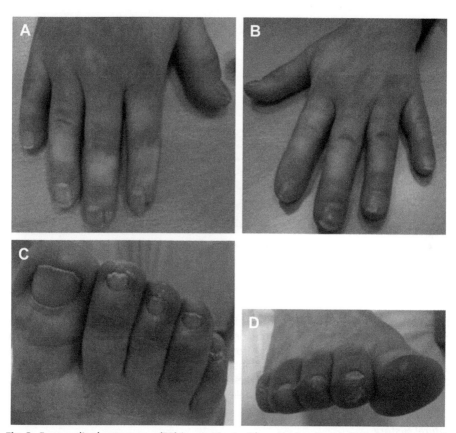

Fig. 3. Raynaud's phenomenon (RP) in a patient with systemic sclerosis (SSc). Note the simultaneous presence of ischemic and cyanotic areas. The asymmetry of the clinical manifestations and the edema of the hands (*A, B*) are indicative of a secondary RP. Feet (*C, D*) demonstrate the presence of nail dystrophy and the outcome of acral ulcer at the level of the second digit (*D*). (*From* Prete M, Fatone MC, Favoino E, et al. Raynaud's phenomenon: from molecular pathogenesis to therapy. Autoimmun Rev 2014;13:657; with permission.)

Histopathology of Skin Biopsies

Skin biopsy is performed only in cases of diagnostic uncertainty. Early in the disease, skin histopathology may illustrate perivascular T lymphocytes/monocytes infiltrates and thickened collagen bundles in the deep dermis.[13] With disease progression, the epidermis atrophies and the dermis accumulates compact hyalinized collagen bundles, fibronectin, and other structural matrix proteins. Late skin lesions demonstrate a paucity of dermal inflammatory cells and capillaries.[14] Moreover, collagen may replace fat cells in the subcutaneous tissue.

Differential Diagnosis

Although the new ACR/EULAR classification system for SSc has an improved sensitivity and specificity compared with the previous 1980 ACR preliminary criteria,[2] with sensitivity of 91% and specificity of 92%, skin thickening is a common feature of several other inflammatory and immune-mediated diseases. The pattern of skin involvement, combined with salient features of the patient's past medical history and exposures, can help to discern the underlying cause of skin thickening

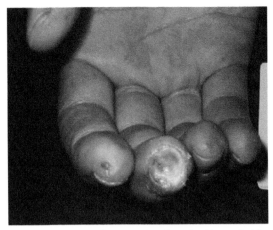

Fig. 4. Digital ulcers in a patient with systemic sclerosis. (*From* Guiducci S, Giacomelli R, Matucci-Cerinic M. Vascular complications of scleroderma. Autoimmun Rev 2007;6:521; with permission.)

(**Table 2**). Notably, the presence of RP is usually absent in SSc mimics (with rare exception in scleromyxedema). Additional diseases, which are not presented in **Table 2**, can have associated skin sclerosis; these conditions are usually diagnosed based on the patient history (eg, amyloidosis, overlap connective tissue diseases, necrobiosis diabeticorum, chronic graft-versus-host disease, sarcoidosis, myxedema, porphyria cutanea tarda, acromegaly), followed by appropriate laboratory testing.

Natural History

Although there is variability in the natural history of SSc skin disease, characteristic patterns are found for DcSSc and LcSSc and are outlined.

Diffuse Cutaneous Involvement

In patients with DcSSc, rapid and intense increases in skin thickening are observed early in the disease course, peaking 1 to 3 years after disease onset.[3] Skin thickening commences distally and progresses proximally to the forearms, arms, and legs, and occasionally the trunk, within several months.[5] The onset of RP typically precedes the development of skin changes by 1 year or less in patients with diffuse skin disease and may even start after the onset of skin thickening.[5]

A single-center, observational study characterized the progression of skin disease in DcSSc patients (n = 826).[15] The authors calculated the skin thickness progression rate (STPR) by dividing the mRSS at the first clinical visit by the duration, in years, from when the patient reported or a physician judged/recorded the onset of skin thickening. The study demonstrated that patients with a rapid STPR (defined as $\geq$40 units/y) had a higher median total skin score and a shorter interval between the onset of skin thickening and their first clinical visit compared with patients with an intermediate (15–40 units/y) or slow (<15 units/y) STPR.[15] Moreover, rapid STPR was found to be an independent predictor of both mortality (odds ratio, 1.72; P = .01) and renal crisis (odds ratio, 2.05; P = .02) within 2 years from first evaluation.[15]

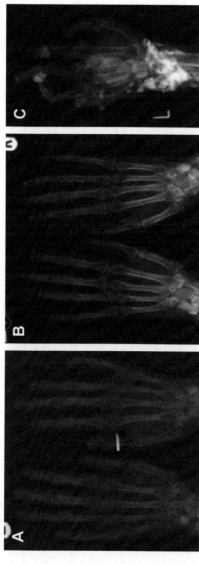

Fig. 5. Calcinosis of the hands in systemic sclerosis with mild (*A*), moderate (*B*), and severe (*C*) involvement. (*From* Chung L, Valenzuela A, Fiorentino D, et al, on behalf of the Scleroderma Clinical Trials Consortium Calcinosis Working Group. Validation of a novel radiographic scoring system for calcinosis affecting the hands of patients with systemic sclerosis. Arthritis Care Res 2015;67(3):427; with permission.)

Table 2
Distinguishing features of systemic sclerosis mimics

Disease	Distribution of Skin Thickening	Appearance	Key Dermal Histopathology	Associated Conditions
Scleromyxedema	Head, neck, upper trunk, forearm, hands, thighs	Waxy, closely spaced papules	Increased mucin, collagen, fibroblasts	Monoclonal gammopathy (especially immunoglobulin G lambda)
Scleroderma	Neck, upper back, shoulders	Erythematous induration	Increased mucin, collagen	Monoclonal gammopathy; diabetes mellitus; postinfectious
Morphea	Localized, linear, deep, or generalized	Erythematous plaque → hyperpigmented or hypopigmented	Increased collagen (no increase in mucin)	None
Nephrogenic systemic sclerosis	Starts distally and spreads proximally (spares face)	Peau d'orange; cobblestone	Increased mucin, collagen, fibroblasts	Renal insufficiency with gadolinium exposure
Eosinophilic fasciitis	Proximal extremities (spares hands, feet)	Rapid swelling → Peau d'orange; groove sign	Increased eosinophils in the deep dermis and fascia	Antecedent vigorous exercise Cytopenias, aplastic anemia

Data from Nashel J, Steen V. Scleroderma mimics. Curr Rheumatol Rep 2012;14:39–46; and Tyndall A, Fistarol S. The differential diagnosis of systemic sclerosis. Curr Opin Rheumatol 2013;25:692–9.

Cutaneous improvement most often occurs first in the areas that were last affected (ie, trunk, abdomen, upper arms).[5] Despite regression of skin thickening in proximal areas, finger and joint contractures often persist. Improvements in skin thickening have been associated with improved survival in observational cohorts.[16]

Limited Cutaneous Involvement

In general, the rate of STPR is much slower in LcSSc compared with DcSSc.[17] The onset of RP typically precedes the development of skin changes by several years (occasionally decades) in patients with LcSSc.[5] In the early stages of limited disease, puffy hands predominate. As skin thickening progresses, involvement remains confined to the hands, distal forearms, lower legs, and feet, with or without the face. Late-stage LcSSc is typically characterized by no further skin thickening, but is often associated with additional skin changes, including the development of subcutaneous calcinosis, digital tip ischemia, and telangiectasias.[5] Occasionally, palpable purpura can occur when vasculitis develops. Visceral involvement can and does occur, particularly in the gastrointestinal tract and lungs, but it tends to occur later in the disease.[5]

MANAGEMENT OF SKIN SCLEROSIS
Existing Therapies

Methotrexate
A folate analog originally designed to inhibit dihydrofolate reductase, methotrexate (MTX) has been used extensively for the treatment of rheumatoid arthritis since the 1950s. Concerns regarding pulmonary fibrosis may have hindered the introduction of MTX into the SSc clinical research arena. However, encouraging observations from small, uncontrolled studies in the early 1990s[18–20] led to the development of the first randomized, controlled trial (RCT) of MTX in SSc.[21] In this study of patients with both LcSSc (n = 18) and DcSSc (n = 11), there was a trend for an improvement in skin score in patients treated with weekly MTX at 24 weeks ($P = .06$).[21]

A study of 71 patients with early (<3 years disease duration) DcSSc found that between-group differences for changes in skin score at 12 months favored MTX (change in mRSS was -4.3 in the MTX group vs 1.8 in the placebo group [$P<.009$]).[22] However, this study observed the greatest difference in skin scores between the treatment and placebo groups early in the trial (3 months), and the difference decreased with time. A follow-up analysis of these data using a Bayesian statistical approach demonstrated that MTX had a 90.4% probability of improving skin scores in DcSSc.[23]

The EULAR and the European Scleroderma Trials and Research Group (EUSTAR)[24] have recommended that MTX be considered for treatment of sclerosis in early DcSSc. Safety concerns regarding the development of pulmonary fibrosis with MTX use have not been substantiated, although this issue has not been formally and systematically addressed.

Practice tip: Consider using MTX for early diffuse skin disease in SSc.

Cyclophosphamide
Although cyclophosphamide (CYC) has been predominantly studied in the context of SSc-associated interstitial lung disease (ILD), this alkylating agent may have beneficial effects on SSc-cutaneous sclerosis. For example, in the Scleroderma Lung Study (SLS) I, 158 SSc patients with both LcSSc and DcSSc (<7 years from first non-Raynaud's SSc manifestation), were randomized to treatment with daily

oral CYC (up to 2 mg/kg per day) for 12 months versus placebo.[25] Patients with DcSSc randomized to CYC had an improvement in mRSS of -5.3 at 12 months, whereas the patients in the placebo group had an improvement in mRSS of only -1.7 at 12 months (P = .008). For an additional 6 months after stopping the CYC, skin continued to improve. However, beyond that point, skin rapidly worsened so that by 24 months, there was no difference between CYC and placebo (P = .23).[26] Although not proven, it is tempting to allow patients to use CYC for a year, stop the drug for some period of time and then consider retreating when skin worsens (personal opinion).

The potential benefits of CYC in treating DcSSc are tempered by the plethora of adverse effects associated with CYC use. One of the most potent immunosuppressive drugs used in rheumatology, CYC can cause serious and life-threatening adverse effects. However, examination of the SLS I study comparing CYC with placebo, showed only increases in neutropenia and infections with very few cases of hematuria or other significant adverse effects during the 12-month trial (including no differences in death or cancer).[27] Notably, this study did not follow patients over then long term, so it did not address the incidence of long-term cancers, which have been documented when using CYC.[27] Most experts consider using CYC for diffuse cutaneous disease only when ILD is also present.

Practice tip: Consider using CYC for patients with early DcSSc when concurrent, clinically significant ILD is present. It should not be considered as the first drug of choice secondary to its potential toxicities.

Autologous hematopoietic stem cell transplantation

Hematopoietic stem cell transplantation (HSCT) has recently emerged as a potentially effective treatment option for carefully selected patients with progressive DcSSc with a poor prognosis.[28] To date, nearly all experience is with autologous HSCT. Early trials demonstrated the feasibility of autologous HSCT in DcSSc and found a significant reduction in mRSS.[29–31] The improvement in mRSS seems to be sustained based on an observational study of 26 transplanted SSc patients followed for 7 years after HSCT.[32] The Autologous Stem Cell Transplantation International Scleroderma (ASTIS) trial was the first phase III RCT designed to compare the efficacy and safety of autologous HSCT versus monthly intravenous CYC for 12 months.[33] This 29-center European study included 156 patients with DcSSc (<4 years duration) and without serious comorbidities. In the first year, mortality was higher in the HSCT group (8 treatment-related deaths), compared with the CYC group (no treatment-related deaths); however, the HSCT group experienced statistically better event-free survival; events included need for dialysis and need for oxygen, and so on (median follow-up time was 5.8 years).[33] The mean improvement in mRSS from baseline to 24 months was greater in the HSCT group (a decrease of 19.9 in the mRSS) than in the control group (a decrease of 8.8; P<.001).[33] Results of the North American phase III RCT (Scleroderma: Cyclophosphamide Or Transplantation, or SCOT trial) are awaiting publication. Future studies are needed to evaluate long-term potential HSCT-related complications (ie, infertility, secondary autoimmune disease, and malignancy), to determine the appropriate timing of HSCT, and to optimize the patient selection criteria to minimize early HSCT-related mortality.

Practice tip: Consider referral for HSCT in patients with DcSSc with poor prognosis, for whom the duration of nonsevere internal organ involvement is less than 4 years and for whom conventional therapies have failed. This should be considered a third-line therapy only.

Ineffective Therapies

Several RCTs and open-label trials have investigated the efficacy of additional experimental agents for the treatment of skin sclerosis in early stage DcSSc. These agents failed to demonstrate a beneficial effect on skin disease outcomes and/or were not tolerated:

- *N*-Acetylcysteine,[34]
- D-Penicillamine,[35]
- Anti-transforming growth factor β-1 antibody,[36]
- Recombinant human relaxin,[37]
- Interferon alpha,[38]
- Imatinib,[39] and
- Bosentan.[40]

Questionable Therapies

These studies demonstrated negative findings:

- Tumor necrosis factor inhibitors,[41,42] and
- Oral type I collagen[43]; post hoc analysis demonstrated cutaneous improvement in patients with late dsSSc.

Experimental Therapies

Advances toward understanding the pathogenesis of SSc-cutaneous sclerosis have augmented the arsenal of candidate therapies for this devastating illness. Diverse molecular targets are presently under preclinical and clinical evaluation.

B-cell target therapies

Previous studies have demonstrated an increased number of B cells in the skin of SSc patients,[44] and that B-cell depletion reduces skin fibrosis in mouse models.[45] To this end, clinical studies have investigated the safety and efficacy of the anti-CD20 antibody, rituximab. Three open-label studies of rituximab in SSc patients,[46–48] one of which showed a significant decrease in hyalinized collagen content and myofibroblast positivity,[46] demonstrated that rituximab may improve the mRSS. These findings indicate that rituximab needs to be further tested in controlled studies.

Interleukin-6

Evidence suggests that the pleiotropic cytokine, interleukin (IL)-6, is overexpressed in the skin of patients with SSc,[49] and may play a unique role in moderating endothelial cell dysfunction and fibrogenesis in this disease.[50] This has led to 2 open-label trials of tocilizumab, the humanized monoclonal antibody to the IL-6 receptor.[51,52] An uncontrolled EUSTAR observational study of 15 SSc patients with arthritis did not show a significant improvement in the mRSS after treatment with tocilizumab after 5 months.[51] However, the primary endpoint for this study was arthritis. Moreover, this study included patients with both LcSSc and DcSSc. An 83-patient, placebo-controlled, multicenter, phase 2 RCT recently demonstrated favorable trends in skin score and lung function at 24 weeks (although the primary skin score endpoint was not met).[53] A fully powered phase 3 trial is clearly needed.

Intravenous immunoglobulin

A paucity of evidence supports the use of intravenous immunoglobulin for SSc.[54] Studies suggest that intravenous immunoglobulin administration is associated with fibrosis resorption in a variety of immune disorders.[55] A small study of 15 patients with both LcSSc and DcSSc demonstrated that monthly intravenous immunoglobulin infusions (2 g/kg infused over a 5-day period for 6, 4, or 3 cycles) was associated with a significant decrease in mRSS of 35% ($P<.001$).[54] Future RCTs are necessary to determine whether this intervention is beneficial.

Mycophenolate mofetil
Mycophenolate mofetil (MMF) is the prodrug to mycophenolic acid, which reversibly inhibits inosine monophosphate dehydrogenase, thereby impairing purine synthesis and lymphocyte proliferation. MMF has both antifibrotic and immunomodulatory effects in animals and may improve skin sclerosis in DcSSc.[56] Thus far, only open-label trials or observational studies have been published. Two small, open-label trials showed significant skin improvements in DcSSc.[57,58] The Medoza and colleagues[58] study also found a decrease in the abundance and thickness of collagen bundles in the dermis in 3 patients who underwent histopathological skin examination before and after MMF treatment.

Although no RCT of MMF in SSc have been published, a large, double-blind multi-center, RCT comparing CYC with MMF for the treatment of SSc-ILD (SLS II) is under-way and the results of this study should be available in the second or third quarter of 2015; it will undoubtedly include an examination of the skin. At present, MMF is considered a second-line medication for the treatment of DcSSc.[59]

Hyperimmune caprine serum
Hyperimmune caprine serum (AIMSPRO, Anti-inflammatory IMmuno -Suppressive PROduct) is a novel, therapeutic product that primarily contains caprine immunoglo-bulins, but also consists of cytokines IL-4 and IL-10, propiomelanocortin, arginine vasopressin, β-endorphin, and corticotropin-releasing factor. In a very small (n = 20), double-blind, placebo-controlled, parallel group study of late-stage DcSSc patients, subjects were randomized to receive 1 mL of AIMSPRO or placebo subcu-taneously twice weekly for 6 months.[60] The mean mRSS decreased by only 1.4 units in the AIMSPRO group, whereas it increased by 2.1 units in the placebo group. A secondary responder analysis revealed a clinically meaningful improvement in mRSS at 26 weeks in 5 actively treated patients (50%) compared with 1 (10%) in the control group ($P = .06$). No additional trials of AIMSPRO in SSc have been pub-lished to date.

MANAGEMENT OF NONSCLEROTIC SKIN MANIFESTATIONS
Raynaud's Phenomenon

Given that RP is a universal feature of SSc, providers for SSc patients need to be adept at managing this condition. The first step of management is to educate the patient to avoid/minimize common precipitating factors, such as cold temperature, stress, and nicotine. Medications associated with RP (ie, ergot derivatives, β-blockers) should be discontinued if clinically possible.

After these general measures are taken, a consensus- and data-based set of rec-ommendations from EULAR[24] suggested that first-line pharmacologic therapy should consist of a calcium channel blocker. Intravenous iloprost, a prostacyclin analog, administered over 3 to 5 days, is indicated in patients for whom calcium channel blocker are ineffective.[24] Although 2 RCTs comparing intravenous iloprost with nifedipine demonstrated slight superiority of iloprost for RP symptoms in SSc,[61,62] oral iloprost was ineffective in a double-blind, controlled, multicenter RCT.[63]

Phosphodiesterase type 5 inhibitors (ie, sildenafil, tadalafil, vardenafil) have been associated with improvement in RP symptoms in several placebo-controlled trials[64–66] and can be used as add-on therapy to calcium channel blockers.

Additional therapies for RP (with weaker evidence) include:

- Glyceryl trinitrate patch,[67]
- Angiotensin II receptor antagonists, such as losartan,[68]
- Alpha-adrenergic blockers, such as prazosin,[69]
- Selective serotonin reuptake inhibitor, such as fluoxetine,[70] and
- Botulinum toxin.[71]

Ischemic Ulceration

While the etiology of ischemic ulcerations is multifactorial and often depends on the ulcer location, DU are in part attributable to persistent vasospasm from RP, plus an underlying vasculopathy associated with SSc.[72,73] In addition to avoiding precipitating factors, bosentan may reduce the number of new ulcerations, especially in patients with an increased number of ulcers.[74]

In patients with severe DU, short-term (ie, 5 days) parenteral prostacyclin-based therapy is often indicated. Both iloprost and treprostinil administration are associated reduced healing time and formation of new DU.[74,75] Moreover, small, single studies (both controlled and uncontrolled) have demonstrated that hyperbaric oxygen,[76] vitamin E,[77] and statins[78] may each reduce healing time of DU.

Comorbid conditions associated with ulcers, such as infection or possible thrombosis, require prompt and aggressive treatment. Ulcers are often exquisitely painful, and patients require appropriate analgesic therapy. Finally, surgical intervention (ie, microsurgical revascularization, digital arterial reconstruction, peripheral digital sympathectomy) may be indicated for refractory, nonhealing ulcers.[79,80]

Other Nonsclerotic Skin Manifestations

Few RCTs have been performed to address the other nonsclerotic, cutaneous manifestations of SSc. Thus, therapeutic options for these conditions are limited (**Table 3**).

FUTURE CONSIDERATIONS/SUMMARY

Cutaneous involvement is a central feature of SSc, afflicting patients with both LcSSc and DcSSc. Among the many cutaneous SSc manifestations (ie, telangiectasias,

Table 3			
Management of nonsclerotic skin manifestations of systemic sclerosis			
Symptom	**Pharmacologic Approach**	**Physical Treatment**	**Investigational Approaches**
Calcinosis	Topical intralesional corticosteroids Diltazem[a]	Carbon dioxide laser Extracorporeal shock wave lithotripsy Surgery in select cases[b]	Rituximab
Telangiectasia	No evidence	Intense pulsed light; pulse dye laser	Topical calcipotriene
Pigment changes	No evidence	—	Topical calcipotriene Vitamin A derivatives

Please note that the quality of the evidence presented in this table is insufficient to make formal treatment recommendations.

[a] Although some case reports have suggested that diltiazem promotes calcinosis regression,[89] others have found no improvement in calcinosis with this agent.[90]

[b] Surgery is typically reserved for well-demarcated, localized lesions to ameliorate pain or as a last resort in refractory cases.

Data from Refs.[81–88]

calcinosis, hypopigmentation or hyperpigmentation), cutaneous sclerosis and RP affect virtually all patients with SSc. Cutaneous sclerosis, in particular, serves as a major physical and psychological burden for patients. Evidence-based treatment options for DcSSc-cutaneous sclerosis include MTX (often first line), CYC (for patients with concurrent ILD), MMF (for patients who failed MTX), and even HSCT (for patients with early, aggressive, and refractory disease). As our understanding of the pathophysiology of SSc evolves, new experimental therapeutic options are being tested (ie, B cells, IL-6). Future RCTs are needed to evaluate the safety and efficacy of these novel agents and to develop predictors of risk and response.

REFERENCES

1. LeRoy EC, Black C, Fleischmajer R, et al. Scleroderma (systemic sclerosis): classification, subsets and pathogenesis. J Rheumatol 1988;15:202–5.
2. van den Hoogen F, Khanna D, Fransen J, et al. 2013 classification criteria for systemic sclerosis: an American College of Rheumatology/European League against Rheumatism collaborative initiative. Arthritis Rheum 2013;65:2737–47.
3. Clements PJ, Medsger TA Jr, Feghali CA. Cutaneous involvement in systemic sclerosis. In: Clements PJ, Furst DE, editors. Systemic sclerosis. 2nd edition. New York: Lippincott Williams and Wilkins; 2004. p. 129–50.
4. Steen VD, Ziegler GL, Rodnan GP, et al. Clinical and laboratory associations of anticentromere antibody in patients with progressive systemic sclerosis. Arthritis Rheum 1984;27:125–31.
5. Medsgar TA Jr. Natural history of systemic sclerosis and the assessment of disease activity, severity, functional status, and psychologic well-being. Rheum Dis Clin North Am 2003;29:255–73.
6. Reveille JD, Fischbach M, McNearney T, et al. Systemic sclerosis in 3 US ethnic groups: a comparison of clinical, sociodemographic, serologic, and immunogenetic determinants. Semin Arthritis Rheum 2001;30:332–46.
7. Herrick AL, Oogarah PK, Freemont AJ, et al. Vasculitis in patients with systemic sclerosis and severe digital ischaemia requiring amputation. Ann Rheum Dis 1994;53:323–6.
8. Furst DE, Clements PJ, Steen VD, et al. The modified Rodnan skin score is an accurate reflection of skin biopsy thickness in systemic sclerosis. J Rheumatol 1998;25:84–8.
9. Clements PJ, Lachenbruch PA, Ng SC, et al. Skin score. A semiquantitative measure of cutaneous involvement that improves prediction of prognosis in systemic sclerosis. Arthritis Rheum 1990;33:1256–63.
10. Khanna D, Furst DE, Hays RD, et al. Minimally important difference in diffuse systemic sclerosis: results from the D-penicillamine study. Ann Rheum Dis 2006;65:1325–9.
11. Bendeck SE, Jacobe HT. Ultrasound as an outcome measure to assess disease activity in disorders of skin thickening: an example of the use of radiologic technique to assess skin disease. Dermatol Ther 2007;20:86–92.
12. Smith V, Riccieri V, Pizzorni C, et al. Nailfold capillaroscopy for prediction of novel future severe organ involvement in systemic sclerosis. J Rheumatol 2013;40:2023–8.
13. Torres JE, Sanchez JL. Histopathological differentiation between localized and systemic sclerosis. Am J Dermatopathol 1998;20:242–5.
14. Prescott RJ, Freemont AJ, Jones CJ, et al. Sequential dermal microvascular and perivascular changes in the development of scleroderma. J Pathol 1992;166:255–63.

15. Domsic RT, Rodriguez-Reyna T, Lucas M, et al. Skin thickness progression rate: a predictor of mortality and early internal organ involvement in diffuse scleroderma. Ann Rheum Dis 2011;70:104–9.
16. Steen VD, Medsger TA Jr. Improvement in skin thickening in systemic sclerosis associated with improved survival. Arthritis Rheum 2001;44:2828–35.
17. Krieg T, Takehara K. Skin disease: a cardinal feature of systemic sclerosis. Rheumatology (Oxford) 2009;48:14–8.
18. Bode BY, Yocum DE, Gall EP, et al. Methotrexate (MTX) in scleroderma: experience in ten patients. Arthritis Rheum 1990;33(Suppl 9):S66.
19. van den Hoogen FH, Boerbooms AM, van de Putte LB, et al. Low dose methotrexate treatment in systemic sclerosis. J Rheumatol 1991;18:1763–4.
20. Seibold JR, McCloskey DA, Furst DE. Pilot trial of methotrexate (MTX) in treatment of early diffuse scleroderma. Arthritis Rheum 1994;37(Suppl 16):R35.
21. van den Hoogen FH, Boerbooms AM, Swaak AJ, et al. Comparison of methotrexate with placebo in the treatment of systemic sclerosis: a 24 week randomized double-blind trial, followed by a 24 week observational trial. Br J Rheumatol 1996;35:364–72.
22. Pope JE, Bellamy N, Seibold JR, et al. A randomized, controlled trial of methotrexate versus placebo in early diffuse scleroderma. Arthritis Rheum 2001;44:1351–8.
23. Johnson SR, Feldman BM, Pope JE, et al. Shifting our thinking about uncommon disease trials: the case of methotrexate in scleroderma. J Rheumatol 2009;36:323–9.
24. Kowal-Bielecka O, Landewé R, Avouac J, et al. EULAR recommendations for the treatment of systemic sclerosis: a report from the EULAR Scleroderma Trials and Research group (EUSTAR). Ann Rheum Dis 2009;68:620–8.
25. Tashkin DP, Elashoff R, Clements PJ, et al, Scleroderma Lung Study Research Group. Cyclophosphamide versus placebo in scleroderma lung disease. N Engl J Med 2006;354:2655–66.
26. Tashkin DP, Elashoff R, Clements PJ, et al, Scleroderma Lung Study Research Group. Effects of 1-year treatment with cyclophosphamide on outcomes at 2 years in scleroderma lung disease. Am J Respir Crit Care Med 2007;176:1026–34.
27. Furst DE, Tseng CH, Clements PJ, et al. Adverse events during the Scleroderma Lung Study. Am J Med 2011;124:459–67.
28. Naraghi K, van Laar JM. Updated on stem cell transplantation for systemic sclerosis: recent trial results. Curr Rheumatol Rep 2013;15:326.
29. Binks M, Passweg JR, Furst D, et al. Phase I/II trial of autologous stem cell transplantation in systemic sclerosis: procedure related mortality and impact on skin disease. Ann Rheum Dis 2001;60:577–84.
30. Farge D, Passweg J, van Laar JM, et al, EBMT/EULAR Registry. Autologous stem cell transplantation in the treatment of systemic sclerosis. Ann Rheum Dis 2004;63:974–81.
31. Nash RA, McSweeney PA, Nelson JL, et al. Allogeneic marrow transplantation in patients with severe systemic sclerosis: resolution of dermal fibrosis. Arthritis Rheum 2006;54:1982–6.
32. Vonk MC, Marjanovic Z, van den Hoogen FH, et al. Long-term follow-up results after autologous haematopoietic stem cell transplantation for severe systemic sclerosis. Ann Rheum Dis 2008;67:98–104.
33. van Laar JM, Farge D, Sont JK, et al. Autologous hematopoietic stem cell transplantation vs intravenous pulse cyclophosphamide in diffuse cutaneous systemic sclerosis: a randomized clinical trial. JAMA 2014;311:2490–8.

34. Furst DE, Clements PJ, Harris R, et al. Measurement of clinical change in progressive systemic sclerosis: a 1 year double-blind placebo-controlled trial of N-acetylcysteine. Ann Rheum Dis 1979;38:356–61.

35. Clements PJ, Furst DE, Wong WK, et al. High-dose versus low-dose D-penicillamine in early diffuse systemic sclerosis: analysis of a two-year, double-blind, randomized, controlled clinical trial. Arthritis Rheum 1999;42:1194–203.

36. Denton CP, Merkel PA, Furst DE, et al. Recombinant human anti-transforming growth factor beta1 antibody therapy in systemic sclerosis: a multi-center, randomized, placebo-controlled phase I/II trial of CAT-192. Arthritis Rheum 2007; 56:323–33.

37. Khanna D, Clements PJ, Furst DE, et al. Recombinant human relaxin in the treatment of systemic sclerosis with diffuse cutaneous involvement: a randomized, double-blind, placebo-controlled trial. Arthritis Rheum 2009;60:1102–11.

38. Black CM, Silman AJ, Herrick AI, et al. Interferon-alpha does not improve outcome at one year in patients with diffuse cutaneous scleroderma: results of a randomized, double-blind, placebo-controlled trial. Arthritis Rheum 1999;42: 299–305.

39. Pope J, McBain D, Petrlich L, et al. Imatinib in active diffuse cutaneous systemic sclerosis: Results of a six-month, randomized, double-blind, placebo-controlled, proof-of-concept pilot study at a single center. Arthritis Rheum 2011;63:3547–51.

40. Seibold JR, Denton CP, Furst DE, et al. Randomized, prospective, placebo-controlled trial of bosentan in interstitial lung disease secondary to systemic sclerosis. Arthritis Rheum 2010;62:2101–8.

41. Denton CP, Engelhart M, Tvede N, et al. An open-label pilot study of infliximab therapy in diffuse cutaneous systemic sclerosis. Ann Rheum Dis 2009;68:1433–9.

42. Murdaca G, Spano F, Contatore M, et al. Potential use of TNF-α inhibitors in systemic sclerosis. Immunotherapy 2014;6:283–9.

43. Postlethwaite AE, Wong WK, Clements P, et al. A multicenter, randomized, double-blind, placebo-controlled trial of oral type I collagen treatment in patients with diffuse cutaneous systemic sclerosis: I. Oral type I collagen does not improve skin in all patients, but may improve skin in late-phase disease. Arthritis Rheum 2008;58:1810–22.

44. Whitfield ML, Finlay DR, Murray JI, et al. Systemic and cell type-specific gene expression patterns in scleroderma skin. Proc Natl Acad Sci U S A 2003;100: 12319–24.

45. Hasegawa M, Hamaguchi Y, Yanaba K, et al. B-lymphocyte depletion reduces skin fibrosis and autoimmunity in the tight-skin mouse model for systemic sclerosis. Am J Pathol 2006;169:954–66.

46. Smith V, Van Praet JT, Vandooren B, et al. Rituximab in diffuse cutaneous systemic sclerosis: an open-label clinical and histopathological study. Ann Rheum Dis 2010;69:193–7.

47. Jordan S, Distler JH, Maurer B, et al, on behalf of the EUSTAR Rituximab Study Group. Effects and safety of rituximab in systemic sclerosis: an analysis from the European Scleroderma Trial and Research (EUSTAR) group. Ann Rheum Dis 2014;74:1188–94.

48. Daoussis D, Liossis SN, Athanassios C, et al. Experience with rituximab in scleroderma: results from a 1-year, proof-of-principle study. Rheumatology (Oxford) 2010;49:271–80.

49. Scala E, Pallotta S, Frezzolini A, et al. Cytokine and chemokine levels in systemic sclerosis: relationship with cutaneous and internal organ involvement. Clin Exp Immunol 2004;138:540–6.

50. Khan K, Xu S, Nihtyanova S, et al. Clinical and pathological significance of inter-leukin 6 overexpression in systemic sclerosis. Ann Rheum Dis 2012;71:1235–42.
51. Elhai M, Meunier M, Matucci-Cerinic M, et al, EUSTAR (EULAR Scleroderma Trials and Research group). Outcomes of patients with systemic sclerosis-associated polyarthritis and myopathy treated with tocilizumab or abatacept: a EUSTAR observational study. Ann Rheum Dis 2013;72:1217–20.
52. Shima Y, Kuwahara Y, Murota H, et al. The skin of patients with systemic sclerosis softened during the treatment with anti-IL-6 receptor antibody tocilizumab. Rheumatology (Oxford) 2010;49:2408–12.
53. Khanna D, Denton CP, van Laar JM, et al. Safety and efficacy of subcutaneous tocilizumab in adults with systemic sclerosis: Week 24 data from a Phase 2/3 Trial. Abstract presentation at the American College of Rheumatology Annual Meeting. Boston, November 15–18, 2014.
54. Levy Y, Amital H, Langevitz P, et al. Intravenous immunoglobulin modulates cuta-neous involvement and reduces skin fibrosis in systemic sclerosis: an open-label study. Arthritis Rheum 2004;50:1005–7.
55. Amital H, Rewald E, Levy Y, et al. Fibrosis regression induced by intravenous gammaglobulin treatment. Ann Rheum Dis 2003;62:175–7.
56. Omair M, Alahmadi A, Johnson SR. Safety and effectiveness of mycophenolate in systemic sclerosis: a systemic review [abstract]. Arthritis Rheum 2013;65(Suppl 10):2599.
57. Derk CT, Grace E, Shenin M, et al. A prospective open-label study of mycophe-nolate mofetil for the treatment of diffuse systemic sclerosis. Rheumatology (Oxford) 2009;48:1595–9.
58. Medoza FA, Nagle SJ, Lee JB, et al. A prospective observational study of myco-phenolate mofetil treatment in progressive diffuse cutaneous systemic sclerosis of recent onset. J Rheumatol 2012;39:1241–7.
59. Walker KM, Pope J, participating members of the Scleroderma Clinical Trials Consortium (SCTC), Canadian Scleroderma Research Group (CSRG). Treat-ment of systemic sclerosis complications: what to use when first-line treatment fails–a consensus of systemic sclerosis experts. Semin Arthritis Rheum 2012; 42:42–55.
60. Quillinan NP, McIntosh D, Vernes J, et al. Treatment of diffuse systemic sclerosis with hyperimmune caprine serum (AIMSPRO): a phase II double-blind placebo-controlled trial. Ann Rheum Dis 2014;73:56–61.
61. Rademaker M, Cooke ED, Almond NE, et al. Comparison of intravenous infu-sions of iloprost and oral nifedipine in treatment of Raynaud's phenomenon in patients with systemic sclerosis: a double blind randomised study. BMJ 1989; 298:561–4.
62. Scorza R, Caronni M, Mascagni B, et al. Effects of long-term cyclic iloprost ther-apy in systemic sclerosis with Raynaud's phenomenon. A randomized, controlled study. Clin Exp Rheumatol 2001;19:503–8.
63. Wigley FM, Korn JH, Csuka ME, et al. Oral iloprost treatment in patients with Ray-naud's phenomenon secondary to systemic sclerosis: a multicenter, placebo-controlled, double-blind study. Arthritis Rheum 1998;41:670–7.
64. Shenoy PD, Kumar S, Jha LK, et al. Efficacy of tadalafil in secondary Raynaud's phenomenon resistant to vasodilator therapy: a double-blind randomized cross-over trial. Rheumatology (Oxford) 2010;49:2420–8.
65. Herrick AL, van den Hoogen F, Gabrielli A, et al. Modified-release sildenafil re-duces Raynaud's phenomenon attack frequency in limited cutaneous systemic sclerosis. Arthritis Rheum 2011;63:775–82.

66. Caglayan E, Axmann S, Hellmich M, et al. Vardenafil for the treatment of Raynaud phenomenon: a randomized, double-blind, placebo-controlled crossover study. Arch Intern Med 2012;172:1182–4.

67. Chung L, Shapiro L, Fiorentino D, et al. MQX-503, a novel formulation of nitroglycerin, improves the severity of Raynaud's phenomenon: a randomized, controlled trial. Arthritis Rheum 2009;60:870–7.

68. Dziadzio M, Denton CP, Smith R, et al. Losartan therapy for Raynaud's phenomenon and scleroderma: clinical and biochemical findings in a fifteen-week, randomized, parallel-group, controlled trial. Arthritis Rheum 1999;42:2646–55.

69. Pope J, Fenlon D, Thompson A, et al. Prazosin for Raynaud's phenomenon in progressive systemic sclerosis. Cochrane Database Syst Rev 2000;(2):CD000956.

70. Coleiro B, Marshall SE, Denton CP, et al. Treatment of Raynaud's phenomenon with the selective serotonin reuptake inhibitor fluoxetine. Rheumatology (Oxford) 2001;40:1038–43.

71. Uppal L, Dhaliwal K, Butler PE. A prospective study of the use of botulinum toxin injections in the treatment of Raynaud's syndrome associated with scleroderma. J Hand Surg Eur Vol 2014;39:876–80.

72. Galluccio F, Matucci-Cerinic M. Two faces of the same coin: Raynaud's phenomenon and digital ulcers in systemic sclerosis. Autoimmun Rev 2011;10:241–3.

73. Matucci-Cerinic M, Denton CP, Furst DE, et al. Bosentan treatment of digital ulcers related to systemic sclerosis: results from the RAPIDS-2 randomised, double-blind, placebo-controlled trial. Ann Rheum Dis 2011;70:32–8.

74. Wigley FM, Seibold JR, Wise RA, et al. Intravenous iloprost treatment of Raynaud's phenomenon and ischemic ulcers secondary to systemic sclerosis. J Rheumatol 1992;19:1407–14.

75. Seibold JR, Wigley FM, Schiopu E, et al. Digital ischemic ulcers in scleroderma treated with oral treprostinil diethanolamine: a randomized, double-blind, placebo-controlled, multicenter study [abstract]. Arthritis Rheum 2011;63(Suppl):S968.

76. Markus YM, Bell MJ, Evans AW. Ischemic scleroderma wounds successfully treated with hyperbaric oxygen therapy. J Rheumatol 2006;33:1694–6.

77. Fiori G, Galluccio F, Braschi F, et al. Vitamin E gel reduces time of healing of digital ulcers in systemic sclerosis. Clin Exp Rheumatol 2009;27:51–4.

78. Abou-Raya A, Abou-Raya S, Helmii M. Statins: potentially useful in therapy of systemic sclerosis-related Raynaud's phenomenon and digital ulcers. J Rheumatol 2008;35:1801–8.

79. Wasserman A, Brahn E. Systemic sclerosis: bilateral improvement of Raynaud's phenomenon with unilateral digital sympathectomy. Semin Arthritis Rheum 2010;40:137–46.

80. Tomaino MM, Goitz RJ, Medsger TA. Surgery for ischemic pain and Raynaud's phenomenon in scleroderma: a description of treatment protocol and evaluation of results. Microsurgery 2001;21:75–9.

81. Hazen PG, Walker AE, Carney JF, et al. Cutaneous calcinosis of scleroderma. Successful treatment with intralesional adrenal steroids. Arch Dermatol 1982;118:366–7.

82. Bottomley WW, Goodfield MJ, Sheehan-Dare RA. Digital calcification in systemic sclerosis: effective treatment with good tissue preservation using the carbon dioxide laser. Br J Dermatol 1996;135:302–4.

83. Sultan-Bichat N, Menard J, Perceau G, et al. Treatment of calcinosis cutis by extracorporeal shock-wave lithotripsy. J Am Acad Dermatol 2012;66:424–9.

84. Merlino G, Germano S, Carlucci S. Surgical management of digital calcinosis in CREST syndrome. Aesthetic Plast Surg 2013;37:1214–9.

85. Dinsdale G, Murray A, Moore T, et al. A comparison of intense pulsed light and laser treatment of telangiectases in patients with systemic sclerosis: a within-subject randomized trial. Rheumatology (Oxford) 2014;53:1422–30.
86. Daoussis D, Antonopoulos I, Liossis SN, et al. Treatment of systemic sclerosis-associated calcinosis: a case report of rituximab-induced regression of CREST-related calcinosis and review of the literature. Semin Arthritis Rheum 2012;41: 822–9.
87. Cunningham BB, Landells ID, Langman C, et al. Topical calcipotriene for morphea/linear scleroderma. J Am Acad Dermatol 1998;39:211–5.
88. Shima Y, Yamamoto Y, Ikeda T, et al. A patient with localized scleroderma successfully treated with etretinate. Case Rep Dermatol 2014;6:200–6.
89. Palmieri GM, Sebes JI, Aelion JA, et al. Treatment of calcinosis with diltiazem. Arthritis Rheum 1995;38:1646–54.
90. Vayssairat M, Hidouche D, Abdoucheli-Baudot N, et al. Clinical significance of subcutaneous calcinosis in patients with systemic sclerosis. Does diltiazem induce its regression? Ann Rheum Dis 1998;57:252–4.

Management of Raynaud Phenomenon and Digital Ulcers in Scleroderma

Laura Cappelli, MD, Fredrick M. Wigley, MD*

KEYWORDS

- Scleroderma • Raynaud phenomenon • Digital ischemia • Digital ulcer
- Prostacyclin • Calcium channel blocker • Thermoregulatory vessels

KEY POINTS

- The pathophysiology of Raynaud phenomenon (RP) and digital ulcers in scleroderma is complex, involving both vasospasm and structural disease of the vasculature.
- Therapy for RP and digital ulcers should involve both nonpharmacologic and pharmacologic treatments.
- Pharmacologic therapy for RP should include a combination of vasoactive agents that can reverse vasoconstriction and address biological pathways to prevent the progression of the underlying vasculopathy.
- Digital ulcers are a common complication of scleroderma vascular disease that requires both systemic and local tissue therapy.
- Critical digital ischemia is a medical emergency and requires urgent treatment. Multiple modalities are available to reverse an event and prevent digital loss.

BACKGROUND

Raynaud phenomenon (RP) is one of the most common clinical manifestations of scleroderma, experienced by 90% to 98% of patients, usually as the first symptom in the course of the disease (**Box 1, Table 1**).[1] The new 2013 classification criteria of the American College of Rheumatology (ACR)/European League Against Rheumatism (EULAR) now recognizes the importance of RP by including it as a feature to confirm a diagnosis of scleroderma.[2] RP often predates other symptoms and signs by several years, which suggests that the peripheral vasculature is the initial target of the scleroderma disease process.[3] The presence of RP alone is a clinical symptom

Disclosures: The authors have no relevant disclosures.
Division of Rheumatology, Johns Hopkins University School of Medicine, 5200 Eastern Avenue, Suite 4100, Mason F. Lord Building, Center Tower, Baltimore, MD 21224, USA
* Corresponding author. Johns Hopkins University School of Medicine, 5200 Eastern Avenue, Suite 4100, Mason F. Lord Building, Center Tower, Baltimore, MD 21224.
E-mail address: fwig@jhmi.edu

Rheum Dis Clin N Am 41 (2015) 419–438
http://dx.doi.org/10.1016/j.rdc.2015.04.005
0889-857X/15/$ – see front matter © 2015 Elsevier Inc. All rights reserved.
rheumatic.theclinics.com

> **Box 1**
> **Key points for the management of digital ulcers**
>
> - Confirm that it is a digital ischemic ulcer and not another digital lesion
> - Maximize vasodilatation
> - Add other proven medications in addition to vasodilators
> - Do not neglect local therapy
> - Evaluate for and treat superinfection
> - Evaluate for macrovascular disease, which can worsen digital ulcers

that is also a predictor of developing scleroderma. This concept is supported by studies finding that patients with a very early diagnosis of scleroderma already have RP.[4,5] Although a patient presenting with only RP, abnormal nail fold capillaries typical of scleroderma, and the presence of a specific scleroderma-related autoantibody do not meet the new ACR/EULAR criteria, studies do find that almost 80% of such patients develop scleroderma over subsequent years of follow-up.[6,7] A recent survey of anti-nuclear antibodies (ANA)-negative patients with scleroderma who did not have RP found that they often had a malignancy, suggesting that these patients may have a cancer-associated syndrome.[8]

To be diagnosed with RP, patients should experience episodic cold-induced or stress-induced sensitivity associated with pallor or cyanosis of the digits.[9] The pallor or cyanosis that accompanies the ischemic phase of an attack may be followed by erythema as a result of reactive hyperemia. Most patients do not experience all phases of color change: pallor, cyanosis, and erythema. The involvement of digital arteries, along with vasoconstriction of cutaneous arterioles, is responsible for the initial color change of pallor witnessed during RP.[10] When veins dilate and there is pooling of deoxygenated blood, the digits take on a cyanotic appearance. Patients with scleroderma are considered to have secondary RP and are more likely to experience digital ulceration and critical digital ischemia than patients with primary RP.[11] Patients with primary RP are less likely to have involvement of the thumb than patients with scleroderma.[12]

In both primary and secondary RP, there is increased reactivity of the blood vessels to cold and increased sympathetic tone. In vitro studies show that increased sympathetic tone is mediated by an increased expression of alpha-2c adrenergic receptors on smooth muscle of cutaneous arteries.[13] Exposure to cold leads to activation of the Rho/Rho-kinase signaling pathway and increased transport of alpha-2c receptors to the cellular membrane.[14] The translocation of these receptors is associated with increased cellular responsiveness to cold-induced adrenergic signals. Ex vivo studies of scleroderma blood vessel have shown that vascular smooth muscle of the arterioles display a selective increase in alpha2-adrenergic reactivity, suggesting that RP in scleroderma is in part caused by upregulation of the adrenergic receptors.[15] In scleroderma, there is also evidence of dysfunction of the endothelium resulting in an imbalance between vasoconstricting and vasodilatory stimuli.[16] Studies have suggested an overproduction of the vasoconstrictor endothelin-1[17] and an underproduction of the vasodilators nitric oxide and prostacyclin by the endothelial cells is involved RP of the peripheral blood vessels.[18]

In humans, the response of the cutaneous circulation to ambient temperature is critical to maintain a normal core temperature. Thermoregulatory vessels are present in the form of arteriovenous shunts in the microcirculation. These vessels are densely distributed in the globular skin of the digits of the hands and feet, accounting for the capacity to rapidly shunt blood from the surface of the skin to deeper tissues to preserve heat. Linked to the thermoregulatory vessels are arterioles and capillaries that provide tissue oxygenation, metabolism, and nutrition. Normally, nutritional flow is not compromised while the thermoregulatory vessels rapidly respond to cold or warm ambient temperatures. The regulation of these thermoregulatory vessels and nutritional vessels is complex, involving both neuropeptides and sympathetic innervation. In patients with severe RP, cold or sympathetic-induced vasospasm occurs in both the superficial thermoregulatory arteriovenous anastomoses in the skin and in blood vessels responsible for nutritional blood flow,[19,20] whereas in normal control subjects, only flow through thermoregulatory vessels is affected.[20] The nutritional blood flow is more severely disrupted in scleroderma compared with normal individuals and those with primary RP, contributing to the increased severity of attacks in scleroderma and the events of tissue ischemia.[19] The increased compromise to tissues in scleroderma is a result of not only an exaggerated response of the thermoregulatory vessels but also a fibro-occlusive vasculopathy of the larger digital arteries, with disease extending into cutaneous capillaries that are critical for tissue nutrition.

The disparate outcomes in RP secondary to scleroderma and primary RP are related to structural abnormalities in blood vessels that develop with scleroderma. Evidence of this can be seen at the bedside when examining the rewarming phase after an RP event. In RP associated with scleroderma, the hyperemic phase after an ischemic event is dampened and blood flow normalization is dramatically prolonged **(Fig. 1)**.[21,22] Abnormalities also occur in the density and structure of arteries, arterioles, and capillaries in scleroderma. RP in scleroderma therefore is associated with loss of the nutritional vasculature to the digits.[11,23,24] In addition, the larger digital arteries are compromised with occlusive intimal hyperplasia and fibrosis caused by increased deposition of collagen.[25] A histologic study of digital arteries showed a greater than 75% reduction in the lumen diameter in 79% of vessels studied.[25] These vascular changes are not limited to the skin or digital vessels but can take place throughout the microcirculation of the vascular system; especially in organs such as the heart, lung, kidneys, and gastrointestinal tract.

In addition to exaggerated vasospasm and structural changes occurring in RP secondary to scleroderma, microthrombi form in blood vessels, leading to tissue damage. This process is likely related to both platelet activation and impaired fibrinolysis.[26] Markers of platelet activation have been shown to be at increased levels in scleroderma, including thromboxane A2, β-thromboglobulin, serotonin, platelet-derived microparticles, and platelet-derived growth factor.[27] Serum levels of one product of platelet activation, CXCL4 (previously known as platelet factor 4), have recently been shown to correlate with the presence of various manifestations of scleroderma, including pulmonary fibrosis and pulmonary hypertension.[28] This study also showed increasing levels of CXCL4 in patients with RP and antinuclear antibodies compared with those with RP alone; even higher levels were found in early scleroderma.[28] Increased levels of tissue plasminogen activator and von Willebrand factor are seen in the plasma of patients with scleroderma, and there is also a defect in fibrinolysis in these patients.[29,30]

The key concept is that scleroderma involves both abnormal vasoreactivity, as is encountered in primary RP, but in addition patients with scleroderma have structural vascular disease and an increased risk of occlusion from abnormally functioning endothelium, platelet activation, and microthrombi. Therefore, managing RP in scleroderma requires more than just vasodilator therapy.

Table 1
Medication options for RP and digital ulcers

Class of Medication	Mechanism of Action	Specific Drugs	Evidence	Strength of Evidence
Calcium channel blockers	Prevents calcium from entering muscle cells and inducing vasospasm	Nifedipine Nicardipine Amlodipine Felodipine Diltiazem	RCT, meta-analysis	Level 1
PDE-5 inhibitors	Inhibits degradation of cGMP promoting vasodilation by NO	Sildenafil Tadalafil Vardenafil	RCT, meta-analysis	Level 1
Prostacyclins	Directly dilate blood vessels, inhibit platelet aggregation	Epoprostenol Iloprost	RCT	Level 2
Topical nitrate	Stimulates cGMP production causing vasodilation	Glyceryl trinitrate	RCT	Level 2
Endothelin receptor antagonists	Blocks vasoconstrictive effects of endothelin-1	Bosentan Ambrisentan Macitentan	RCT (ulcers only)	Level 2
Statins	Inhibit HMG-CoA reductase reducing LDL cholesterol levels, likely other effects in RP and digital ulcers	Atorvastatin Rosuvastatin Pravastatin	RCT of atorvastatin (RP and ulcers)	Level 2

Angiotensin receptor blockers	Antagonize angiotensin receptors	Losartan Irbesartan Olmesartan	RCT (losartan in RP)	Level 2
Selective serotonin reuptake inhibitors	Prevent serotonin entry into vascular smooth muscle	Fluoxetine Sertraline Paroxetine	RCT for fluoxetine in RP	Level 2
Botulinum toxin	Likely by arterial vasodilation from sympathetic blockade	Botulinum toxin	Case series	Level 3
Immunosuppression	Decreases	Cyclophosphamide Mycophenolate mofetil Azathioprine	No dedicated studies, suggested benefit in 1 study of CYC for other purpose	Level 3
Antiplatelet	Inhibit platelet aggregation	Aspirin Clopidogrel	Negative trials in RP No trials in ulcers	Level 4
Anticoagulation	Inhibit coagulation cascade	Enoxaparin Warfarin	No studies in scleroderma	Level 4
Rho-kinase inhibitors	Prevent vasospasm through Rho-kinase pathway	Fasudil	One small negative trial in RP	Level 4
Guanylate cyclase stimulators	Potentiates vasodilatory effects of nitric oxide	Riociguat	No evidence in RP or ulcers at present	N/A

Abbreviations: cGMP, cyclic guanylyl monophosphate; CYC, cyclophosphamide; HMG-CoA, 3-hydroxy-3-methylglutaryl-coenzyme A; LDL, low-density lipoprotein; PDE-5, phosphodiesterase-5; RCT, randomized controlled trial.

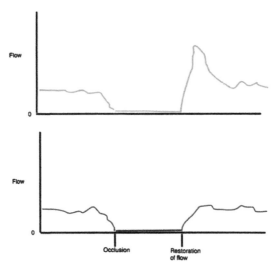

Fig. 1. Doppler-measured blood flow in a digit. The flow is measured at baseline for 5 minutes and then a blood pressure cuff on the proximal finger occludes all flow for 5 minutes. The cuff is then released and reflow is measured. Note the postocclusion hyperemic response in normal individuals (*green*) compared with the abnormal and blunted response to recovery in those with scleroderma who are known to have vascular structural disease of digital arteries (*blue*).

The pathogenesis of scleroderma vascular disease is complex and has been reviewed in several recent articles.[3,17,31] This article focuses on the management of the clinical consequences of scleroderma peripheral vascular disease.

DIGITAL ULCERS

Digital ulcers are ischemic lesions representing end organ damage from the vascular disease of scleroderma. It is defined as an area with a visually discernible depth and a loss of continuity of epithelial coverage. The ischemic ulcer may be denuded or covered by necrotic tissue or scab. The prevalence of digital ulceration in scleroderma has been estimated at 10% to 54%[32–34] and was about 15% in a recently published systematic review of the literature.[35]

Certain subgroups of patients are more likely to develop ulcers. One multivariate analysis showed a correlation between male gender, history of digital ulcers, abnormal nail fold capillaries seen on capillaroscopy, increased erythrocyte sedimentation rate, and the development of new ulcers.[36] Another survey showed younger age of onset of scleroderma, higher finger and hand sclerotic skin score, and presence of interstitial lung disease to be associated with digital ulcers.[34] Patients with antitopoisomerase antibodies may have more complications from digital ischemia and a younger age of onset of digital ulcers.[37] Several investigators have shown an association between advanced nail fold capillary changes and an increased risk of digital ulcers,[38,39] suggesting that abnormal nail fold capillaroscopy pattern is a useful clinical biomarker predicting new ulcer development.

Ischemic digital ulcers are a particularly important clinical problem because they can significantly affect both the quality of life and functional status of patients. One study showed that patients with digital ulcers had significantly decreased hand and wrist mobility, increased hand and wrist disability, and worsened health-related quality of life.[40] The presence of digital ulcers has also been associated with poorer outcomes as measured on a disability index and a scale measuring psychosocial adjustment to illness.[41] Given the associated morbidity, identifying and effectively treating digital ischemic ulcers is critical.

Digital ulcers resulting from ischemia should be differentiated from other digital lesions in scleroderma. A typical digital ischemic ulcer is located on the tip of the finger, on the volar surface, but they can also occur on the extensor surface distal to the interphalangeal joints, particularly around the nail bed (**Fig. 2**).[33] They must be distinguished from dry skin with a fissure, traumatic skin lesions, or ulceration caused by subcutaneous calcinosis. The avascular and fibrotic skin of scleroderma results in a decrease in skin lubrication and progressive dryness with scaling, crusted skin. This process can create a deep fissure (**Fig. 3**) on the fingertip that mimics an ischemic ulcer. Fibrosis in skin and soft tissue structures can also lead to fixed contractures of the fingers, particularly of the proximal interphalangeal joints. These contractures are associated with avascular thin skin that is susceptible to injury and the development of traumatic ulcers (**Fig. 4**). Subcutaneous calcinosis can occur anywhere on the body, but especially on the fingers and other points of trauma. Subcutaneous calcinosis in the finger can rupture through the skin of the fingertip and be confused for an ischemic ulcer (**Fig. 5**). Patients with scleroderma can also develop osteolysis of the distal finger. The loss of bone of the distal phalanx causes a deformity of the fingertip with loss of length of the digit and in some cases a pseudoclubbing of the nail bed (**Fig. 6**). Osteolysis can mimic an ischemic finger because it causes discomfort as bone anatomy is altered. Fissures, trauma, subcutaneous calcinosis, and osteolysis should be considered when evaluating new fingertip lesions in a patient with scleroderma because treatment is different for each type.

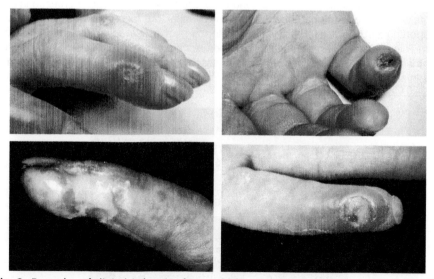

Fig. 2. Examples of digital ischemic ulcers, which are defined as an area with a visually discernible depth and a loss of continuity of epithelial coverage. Ischemic ulcers may be denuded or covered by necrotic tissue or scab, and are located on the distal fingertip or volar-lateral surface.

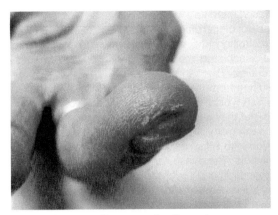

Fig. 3. Dry, fibrotic skin leading to a fissure on the fingertip.

MACROVASCULAR DISEASE IN SCLERODERMA

The understanding of scleroderma as a systemic vasculopathy has increased the recognition of macrovascular disease. Peripheral vascular disease (PVD) was the earliest form of macrovascular disease recognized in scleroderma.[42] PVD can add to the compromise of peripheral blood flow and worsen microvascular manifestations. It may also cause independent issues, including claudication and limb ischemia. Ulnar artery disease is recognized as a common complication in scleroderma that can be shown by an abnormal Allen test. Ulnar artery disease is associated with recurrent digital ulceration in patients with scleroderma.[43] Several studies have also shown that scleroderma is a risk factor for lower extremity PVD manifest by a decreased ankle brachial index.[44–46]

Whether cerebrovascular disease and coronary artery disease are increased in patients with scleroderma had been more controversial, but recent studies present data supporting a true increased risk in the development of arterial sclerosis. A recent study from Taiwan showed an association between ischemic stroke and scleroderma[47] and another from the United Kingdom showed association with increased risk of myocardial infarction, ischemic stroke, and PVD.[48] A meta-analysis also showed a higher

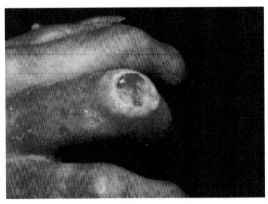

Fig. 4. Traumatic ulcer over a contracture of the proximal interphalangeal joint. These ulcers are caused by thin avascular skin over the contracture that is susceptible to injury.

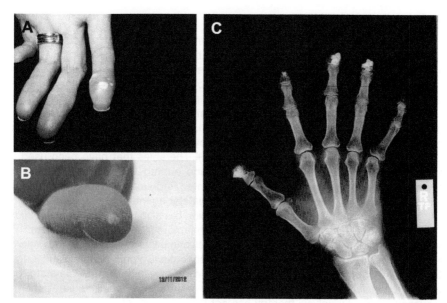

Fig. 5. (*A*) Subcutaneous calcinosis breaking through the skin of the second digit. (*B*) Calcinosis on the tip of a digit mimicking an ischemic ulcer. (*C*) Radiograph shows calcium deposits on the fingertips of a patient with scleroderma.

prevalence of coronary atherosclerosis, PVD, and cerebrovascular calcifications in patients with scleroderma.[49]

Other risk factors for macrovascular disease in scleroderma are similar to those in the general population. Smoking, hyperlipidemia, hypertension, and diabetes can all contribute to atherosclerosis and worsen PVD. Modifying these risk factors is important in the management of macrovascular disease in scleroderma.

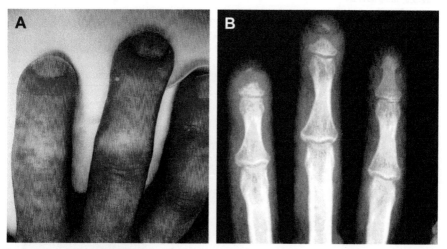

Fig. 6. (*A*) Pseudoclubbing of the distal finger in a patient with scleroderma caused by osteolysis of the distal phalanges (*B*) Loss of distal bone secondary to osteolysis as seen on a plain radiograph of the fingers of the patient seen in *A*.

PRINCIPLES OF MANAGEMENT

Because there is both abnormal vasoreactivity and structural vascular disease causing RP and tissue ischemia in scleroderma, management requires a multitargeted approach. The first intervention should be to prevent vasospasm. Avoiding triggering factors, including cold environments and psychological stress, has a major impact on the disease and management of these factors needs to be emphasized to patients (discussed later). Vasodilator therapy is the first line of drug therapy and should be instituted if nondrug therapy and risk factor avoidance alone are not effective. Preventing further progression of the vascular disease by targeting important biological pathways is now being attempted (discussed later). Therapies that have been used to prevent progression of vascular disease include endothelin receptor antagonists, immunosuppression, statin therapy, antioxidants, Rho-kinase inhibitors, prostacyclins, and angiotensin receptor blockers. Antiplatelet agents are also used not only to decrease microthrombi formation and occlusion but also to prevent vascular injury by inhibiting the release of cytokines and growth factors from activated platelets.[26,50] Aspirin or other platelet inhibitors (eg, clopidogrel) can be used in patients with scleroderma who are at risk for digital ulceration and ischemia. Chronic systemic anticoagulation is not recommended unless there is evidence of a hypercoagulable state, but acute anticoagulation can be considered in severe cases of acute digital ischemia (discussed later). Fibrinolysis therapy has not been formally studied in scleroderma-related vascular disease.

A flow chart of our algorithm for management decisions is shown in **Fig. 7**. Therapy should be added in a stepwise fashion, depending on the individual situation and

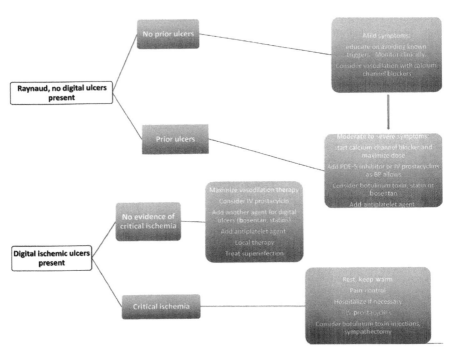

Fig. 7. Management decisions for RP and digital ulcers. BP, blood pressure; IV, intravenous; PDE-5, phosphodiesterase-5.

clinical severity. Specific examples of this decision making are described in the following case presentations.

CASE PRESENTATIONS
Case One

A 31-year-old woman presents to clinic complaining of uncomfortable color changes of her fingers triggered by the cold. The history confirms that she has RP, with attacks since the age of 27 years that have increased in frequency and severity over the last 3 years. She has mild gastrointestinal reflux disease but no clinical or laboratory evidence of interstitial lung disease or pulmonary hypertension. She was recently diagnosed with limited scleroderma when mild sclerodactyly and a positive anticentromere antibody test were found.

She reports increased emotional stress caused by her job as a lawyer, undergoing a divorce, and also having a young child at home. As a result of this stress, she has started smoking 1 pack of cigarettes daily, and she drinks several cups of coffee daily. She has never had a digital ischemic ulcer. Examination is otherwise normal but shows a blood pressure of 100/63 mm Hg, sclerodactyly, abnormal nail fold capillaries, and digital pallor consistent with active RP in the cool examination room. There are no digital ulcers and excellent pulses with no signs of macrovascular disease. Her laboratory data are normal except for a positive ANA test with centromere pattern.

In this patient with no prior digital ulceration, therapeutic goals include improving quality of life and preventing any digital ulcers in the future. The first consideration should be nonpharmacologic therapy. A key aspect of nondrug therapy is educating patients about the goals of the therapy, what is happening to cause the RP, and all aspects of the status and plans to treat the underlying disease; this approach reduces fear and provides a full understanding of what can be done to help achieve ideal management. Patients can acclimate to their daily environments and thus reduce RP events. Patients should be told that, if the core body temperature drops, RP will occur even if the hands and feet are warm. To maintain a normal core body temperature the patient must wear layered warm clothing, including a head cover, and avoiding cold temperatures, especially shifting temperatures at home and in the work environment. In this patient's case, given her anxiety, the use of a selective serotonin reuptake inhibitor (SSRI) is recommended both for her emotional state and to reduce RP events by blocking serotonin uptake by vascular smooth muscle.[51]

An important aspect of this patient's history is her tobacco use. Current smoking was shown to be associated with increased severity of RP and presence of digital ulcerations, and this effect substantially decreased after a year of quitting smoking.[52] Providing counseling and aids for smoking cessation should be part of the therapy for RP.

Whether caffeine should be avoided in RP is not clearly defined. New evidence suggests that caffeine may have vasodilatory effects through the increase of nitric oxide and other mediators acting on the endothelium and vascular smooth muscle cells.[53] Another study, however, showed that caffeine negatively affected the thermogenic response in fingers immersed in cold water, suggesting that it may be detrimental in patients with RP.[54] Until more data are available, we recommend that patients with RP and scleroderma avoid excess caffeine. It is also likely to aggravate gastrointestinal reflux by reducing lower esophageal sphincter tone.

In this young, premenopausal woman, it is unlikely that she would require unopposed estrogen therapy. In older patients, however, this issue may become relevant. There was prior conflicting evidence about this issue. Unopposed estrogen therapy has been associated with increased prevalence of RP in postmenopausal women.[55] In patients with scleroderma, however, it was shown to improve endothelial dysfunction.[56,57] More recently, estrogen has been shown to increase expression of alpha-2c receptors in vitro and to enhance cold-induced vasoconstriction in mouse tail arteries.[58] Taking the more recent evidence of negative vascular effect, we recommend avoiding unopposed estrogen in patients with scleroderma.

Various herbal medications have been used for treatment of RP. For example, *Gingko biloba* has been suggested to be helpful.[59] A recent meta-analysis finds that quality studies of complementary medications are lacking.[60] There is biological plausibility for DSGOST, which is a traditional Chinese therapy used for RP. An in vitro study showed that DSGOST modulated the effects of Rho-kinase and endothelin-1[61]. It is also clear that behavioral therapy such as biofeedback has no solid evidence of effect in scleroderma, and these treatments are not recommended.[60]

If lifestyle modifications and cold avoidance are not sufficient to control the patient's symptoms, vasodilatory therapy should be instituted. Dihydropyridine calcium channel blockers are the first-line therapy. A meta-analysis has documented that these agents provide a definite but modest benefit in scleroderma-associated RP.[62] Options include nifedipine, amlodipine, felodipine, and nicardipine.

In addition to smoking cessation and lifestyle modification, we recommend starting amlodipine 5 mg daily and slowly uptitrating to 10 mg if there is no response in 4 weeks. It can be argued that, if nondrug therapy is effective in improving quality of life, then no drug therapy is needed, but in scleroderma clinicians must consider preventing ischemic events and reducing the risk of systemic vascular disease. Although not proved, some clinicians argue that a calcium channel blocker provides not only a reduction in RP severity but a protection against systemic vascular disease.[63] Concern often arises when patients, like this woman, have a low systemic blood pressure. Usually, patients with systolic blood pressure greater than 90 mm Hg can tolerate a calcium channel blocker. If they have symptomatic hypotension on the calcium channel blocker, 2 alternative options are the use of an SSRI or the local injection of botulinum toxin (Botox). However, more studies are needed to define the benefit of these agents in scleroderma-related RP. In severe cases, periodic infusions of prostacyclin can be considered because blood pressure can be monitored during the infusion and the benefit for RP is reported to last for weeks.[64,65] Infusions of epoprostenol (available in the United States) or iloprost (available in Europe) can be given intermittently.

Other options for vasodilatory therapy include phosphodiesterase-5 (PDE-5) inhibitors like sildenafil or periodic application of topical nitrates. A meta-analysis has shown the benefit of PDE-5 inhibitors in decreasing the frequency and duration of RP attacks.[66] A PDE-5 inhibitor or topical nitrates can be added to a calcium channel blocker in refractory or severe cases or used as first-line therapy if there is contraindication or intolerance to a calcium channel blocker.

The patient was counseled on avoiding triggers of attacks and started on amlodipine 5 mg daily. She was able to quit smoking using resources provided by a smoking cessation hotline. She worked with family, was counseled to help her with social stresses, and she was given an SSRI that helped with anxiety. The frequency and severity of her attacks decreased and no digital ulcers had developed over years of follow-up.

Case Two

A 52-year-old man with a history of long-standing scleroderma with limited skin disease and RP presents with recurrent digital ischemic ulcers of his fingers for the past 2 months. He has been treated with amlodipine 10 mg daily for his RP for 12 months. He is afebrile and well appearing with a blood pressure of 120/60 mm Hg at the clinic visit. Typical ischemic digital ulcers on the tips of 2 fingers on his right hand and 1 finger on his left hand are noted. There is no discharge from the ulcers, and there is no surrounding erythema or swelling. He says the ulcerations are causing him considerable discomfort while performing his activities of daily living, including preventing him from typing on a computer at work.

First, the patient should be counseled about avoiding risk factors for RP, as discussed earlier. Even though he has coped with scleroderma for a long time, the importance of nondrug therapy and lifestyle factors should be reiterated. We recommend that he take days off work to reduce trauma to his fingers and allow him to avoid cold and stress. This nondrug management is a major factor to allow ulcers to heal. He has been started on first-line vasodilatory therapy and is still having ulcerations. One approach is to increase his calcium channel blocker to the maximally tolerated dose. Usually doses more than 15 mg daily of amlodipine lead to some peripheral edema or a decrease in the systemic blood pressure. Another option is to add a second agent or agents to his regimen. We favor adding an agent when recurrent ulcers occur while on a maximally tolerated calcium channel blocker. As previously discussed, consideration can be given to a PDE-5 inhibitor, local Botox injection, topical nitrates, or intermittent intravenous (IV) prostacyclins. We favor adding a PDE-5 inhibitor such as sildenafil at 20 mg 3 times daily. If signs of acute ischemia are present, then we first use IV prostacyclin and then add the PDE-5 inhibitor.

There has been increased interest in using botulinum toxin for treatment of digital ulcers and digital ischemia in scleroderma. One possible mechanism of action is arterial vasodilation from sympathetic blockade[67] but other mechanisms may be relevant. Several studies show decreased pain and increased healing of digital ulcers.[68-71] Botulinum toxin is not yet covered by insurance, and has not been studied in an adequately sized placebo-controlled clinical trial.

In severe cases of refractory digital ulcers despite medical therapy, sympathectomy can be considered. Digital sympathectomy is preferred to a cervical sympathectomy (discussed later).

Local therapy for the ulcers should also be instituted. The ulcers did not appear infected on examination. In ulcers that are infected, we prefer to use oral systemic antibiotics. *Staphylococcus aureus* is the most common pathogen observed in infection of digital ulcers in scleroderma, but gram-negative intestinal bacteria like *Escherichia coli* have been reported.[72] Therefore, first-line therapy for an infected ulcer should cover *Staphylococcus* and *Streptococcus* species and potentially some enteric bacteria. For this we recommend cephalexin or clindamycin. If there is purulence, the antibiotic chosen should cover methicillin-resistant *S aureus*. Trimethoprim/sulfamethoxazole or clindamycin could be used for oral antibiotic therapy. Deeper soft tissue infections can occur and can be challenging to diagnose. Imaging of the digits may be misleading because other entities, like osteolysis, can have a similar appearance to osteomyelitis on imaging. One series in which osteomyelitis was diagnosed based on clinical, laboratory, and imaging findings showed a prevalence of 42% in infected ulcers.[73] If osteomyelitis is suspected, longer therapy with IV antibiotics is required. Infectious disease consultation would be warranted in this setting.

Keeping the ulcers clean and protected from trauma is most important for successful healing to occur. The ulcers should be washed with soap and water twice a day and, for protection, covered with a dressing. A topical antibiotic like mupirocin (2% cream) should be applied to the ulcers while they are still moist or alternatively a dressing with antibacterial properties, like silver colloid, can be used. Once the ulcers have become dry and keratotic, topical antibiotics can be stopped. At this stage, allowing the crusted ulcer to heal without application of topical medications improves outcome. We usually see ulcer healing with this approach in 6 to 9 weeks.

Debridement may be necessary if there is surrounding necrotic tissue, but this should be undertaken with care given that avascular skin is present. Digital ulcers can be extremely painful. We recommend pain control with topical lidocaine (eg, EMLA Cream [lidocaine 2.5% and prilocaine 2.5%]) around the ulcer (not in the wound), nonsteroidal antiinflammatory drugs (eg, ibuprofen 600 mg every 8 hours), and/or low-dose opioids (eg, oxycodone 5 mg every 6 hours if needed). Widespread digital pain that goes beyond the area of the wound is a sign of ongoing ischemia to the digit with persistent vasospasm, vessel occlusion, or associated macrovascular disease that needs immediate attention (discussed later).

Local wound care is equally important in other causes of scleroderma-related digital lesions, such as traumatic ulcers and areas of subcutaneous calcinosis. We recommend the same methods of local therapy and treatment of superinfection for these lesions as for digital ischemic ulcers. Vasodilation therapy to address the underlying vascular disease and improve digital blood flow is important but is not as helpful in cases of calcinosis or at sites of traumatic ulcers. Calcinosis may require surgical debridement if associated with nonhealing wounds. Protection of fingers at sites of contractures is most important to prevent reoccurrences of traumatic ulcers. We use a gel-coated cushioned sleeve or, in severe contractures, surgical correction to straighten the finger.

Prevention of further ulcers should focus on addressing potential biological pathways beyond abnormal vasoreactivity that may contribute to scleroderma vascular disease. Endothelin receptor antagonists have been studied for treatment of digital ulceration and have been shown to prevent development of new ulcers. Bosentan has been studied in 2 randomized placebo-controlled trials.[74,75] Ambrisentan, in a smaller number of patients, has been shown to decrease digital ulcer burden.[76,77] A clinical trial of macitentan, a new generation of endothelin receptor antagonists, was recently discontinued and the final report is awaited.

Other medications that may offer vascular protection in scleroderma include statins and prostacyclins. Statins have been shown in a small trial to decrease the number of new ulcers in patients with scleroderma.[78] The mechanism behind their vascular protection is likely a combination of mobilizing endothelial progenitor cells; improving endothelial function; and antioxidant, antiinflammatory, and antifibrotic properties.[79,80] In addition to their vasodilatory properties, prostacyclins may also have disease-modifying effects in scleroderma vascular disease. The beneficial clinical effects of iloprost last for weeks after the infusion, as does the positive influence on biomarkers of vascular disease.[81]

Riociguat, a soluble guanylate cyclase stimulator, was recently shown to be effective for pulmonary arterial hypertension.[82] It is soon to be tested for RP or digital ulcerations in scleroderma.

Antiplatelet therapy has been studied in RP with no good evidence of benefit. However, the studies to date are small and ideal dosages of various drug options are not defined. There is a strong biological reason to use antiplatelet therapy, as recently reviewed.[26] We recommend using antiplatelet therapy with low-dose aspirin (81 mg daily) if no contraindications are present.

In this patient, we added sildenafil to his vasodilatory regimen. He also began atorvastatin. He was seen at 6-week intervals to evaluate progress. When ulcers persisted, intermittent monthly infusions of epoprostenol were instituted, which ultimately led to healing. No new ulcers have occurred over a year of follow-up.

Case Three

A 45-year-old woman with a history of scleroderma presents with a cyanotic, extremely painful left third finger. She has a history of diffuse skin disease, interstitial lung disease, severe RP, and recurrent digital ulcerations, currently managed with amlodipine, aspirin, and rosuvastatin. Physical examination shows ulcers on several fingertips and cyanosis of the distal tip of the right index and third fingers with diminished capillary refill and exquisite tenderness to palpation. There is no area of gangrene (**Fig. 8**).

Critical digital ischemia is a medical emergency and should be treated quickly and aggressively. We recommend having the patient rest in a warm environment, either at home or hospitalized, to maximize blood flow to the affected finger. Vasodilation should be maximized as much as blood pressure can tolerate. In this severe digital ischemia situation with vasodilation therapy failing, we move quickly to the use of IV prostacyclin. In nonacute situations, we administer epoprostenol via a peripheral vein in an outpatient infusion center. Hospitalizing the patient can also be done to allow for continuous therapy for prostacyclins (0.5–2 ng/kg/min for 3 to 5 days). A cohort study showed that 12% of patients required at least 1 hospitalization for administration of IV prostacyclins in an 18-month period.[83] In a pediatric case series of patients with connective tissue disease and ischemic digits, 74% had restoration of digital flow with IV iloprost.[84] Pain control is also important to the management of critical digital ischemia. Uncontrolled pain can increase sympathetic tone and worsen ischemia. Opioids may have a vasoconstricting effect, but we still use low doses to control pain.

In an acute situation, antiplatelet therapy or anticoagulation should be considered. Although there are no studies on anticoagulation in critical digital ischemia, short-term systemic anticoagulation is sensible with the known pathophysiology of digital ischemia. We use IV heparin in cases in which we suspect acute macrovascular occlusion. We usually anticoagulate for 48 to 72 hours with heparin and do not chronically anticoagulate unless there is evidence of an embolic event or a hypercoagulable state. Antiplatelet agents such as aspirin (81 mg by mouth daily) or clopidogrel should be started if there is no contraindication such as active bleeding.

If rest, pain control, and prostacyclins are not controlling the ischemic event, then surgical sympathectomy is considered. Surgical sympathectomy can be effective in

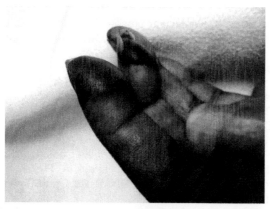

Fig. 8. Example of critical ischemia of the distal second and third digits with no gangrene present.

reversing an acute ischemic crisis when medical therapy is ineffective. The 2 options are proximal (thoracic in the upper extremities) and digital sympathectomy. We no longer use proximal sympathectomy because of the increased morbidity of the procedure and the effectiveness of a distal digital approach. Long-term data for digital sympathectomy are limited but in one systematic review of the literature 18% of patients had a recurrence of ulcers and 14% required amputation.[85] We have used with success botulinum toxin therapy as an alternative to a surgical procedure. Some surgeons are doing digital sympathectomy coupled with local botulinum toxin injections. Clearly, more studies are needed to define the ideal approach.

We admitted the patient to the hospital for monitoring. She was given IV pain medication, the room was warmed, and she was maintained on her aspirin, statin, and amlodipine. She was started on a heparin infusion and IV prostacyclins continuously for vasodilation. Her pain gradually improved but the tip of her finger became gangrenous. We recommended no surgical procedure until natural demarcation occurred to prevent extension of the lesion. Demarcation and autoamputation eventually occurred.

REFERENCES

1. Hudson M, Fritzler MJ, Baron M. Systemic sclerosis: establishing diagnostic criteria. Medicine 2010;89:159–65.
2. van den Hoogen F, Khanna D, Fransen J, et al. 2013 classification criteria for systemic sclerosis: an American College of Rheumatology/European League against Rheumatism collaborative initiative. Arthritis Rheum 2013;65:2737–47.
3. Matucci-Cerinic M, Kahaleh B, Wigley F. Evidence that systemic sclerosis is a vascular disease. Arthritis Rheum 2013;65:1953–62.
4. Avouac J, Fransen J, Walker UA, et al, EUSTAR Group. Preliminary criteria for the very early diagnosis of systemic sclerosis: results of a Delphi Consensus Study from EULAR Scleroderma Trials and Research Group. Ann Rheum Dis 2011;70: 476–81.
5. Valentini G, Marcocia A, Cuomo G, et al. The concept of early systemic sclerosis following 2013 ACR\EULAR criteria for the classification of systemic sclerosis. Curr Rheumatol Rev 2014;10:38–44.
6. LeRoy EC, Medsger TA Jr. Criteria for the classification of early systemic sclerosis. J Rheumatol 2001;28:1573–6.
7. Koenig M, Joyal F, Fritzler MJ, et al. Autoantibodies and microvascular damage are independent predictive factors for the progression of Raynaud's phenomenon to systemic sclerosis: a twenty-year prospective study of 586 patients, with validation of proposed criteria for early systemic sclerosis. Arthritis Rheum 2008;58: 3902–12.
8. Schneeberger D, Tyndall A, Kay J, et al. Systemic sclerosis without antinuclear antibodies or Raynaud's phenomenon: a multicentre study in the prospective EULAR Scleroderma Trials and Research (EUSTAR) database. Rheumatology (Oxford) 2013;52:560–7.
9. Wigley FM. Clinical practice Raynaud's phenomenon. N Engl J Med 2002;347: 1001–8.
10. Flavahan N. Pathophysiological Regulation of the Cutaneous Vascular System in Raynaud's Phenomenon. In: Wigley FM, Herrick A, Flavahan N, editors. Raynaud's phenomenon – A Guide to Pathogenesis and Treatment. New York: Springer; 2014. p. 57–79.
11. Herrick AL. The pathogenesis, diagnosis and treatment of Raynaud phenomenon. Nat Rev Rheumatol 2012;8:469–79.

12. Chikura B, Moore T, Manning J, et al. Thumb involvement in Raynaud's phenomenon as an indicator of underlying connective tissue disease. J Rheumatol 2010; 37:783–6.

13. Chotani MA, Flavahan S, Mitra S, et al. Silent alpha(2C)-adrenergic receptors enable cold-induced vasoconstriction in cutaneous arteries. Am J Physiol Heart Circ Physiol 2000;278:H1075–83.

14. Bailey SR, Eid AH, Mitra S, et al. Rho kinase mediates cold-induced constriction of cutaneous arteries: role of alpha2C-adrenoceptor translocation. Circ Res 2004; 94:1367–74.

15. Flavahan NA, Flavahan S, Liu Q, et al. Increased alpha2-adrenergic constriction of isolated arterioles in diffuse scleroderma. Arthritis Rheum 2000;43:1886–90.

16. Sunderkotter C, Riemekasten G. Pathophysiology and clinical consequences of Raynaud's phenomenon related to systemic sclerosis. Rheumatology (Oxford) 2006;45(Suppl 3):iii33–5.

17. Kahaleh B, Mulligan-Kehoe MJ. Mechanisms of vascular disease. In: Varga J, Denton CP, Wigley FM, editors. Scleroderma: from pathogenesis to comprehensive management. London: Springer Verlag; 2012. p. 227–46.

18. Kahaleh B, Matucci-Cerinic M. Raynaud's phenomenon and scleroderma. Dysregulated neuroendothelial control of vascular tone. Arthritis Rheum 1995;38:1–4.

19. Coffman JD, Cohen AS. Total and capillary fingertip blood flow in Raynaud's phenomenon. N Engl J Med 1971;285:259–63.

20. Carter SA, Dean E, Kroeger EA. Apparent finger systolic pressures during cooling in patients with Raynaud's syndrome. Circulation 1988;77:988–96.

21. Wigley FM, Wise RA, Mikdashi J, et al. The post-occlusive hyperemic response in patients with systemic sclerosis. Arthritis Rheum 1990;33:1620–5.

22. Gaillard-Bigot F, Roustit M, Blaise S, et al. Abnormal amplitude and kinetics of digital postocclusive reactive hyperemia in systemic sclerosis. Microvasc Res 2014;94:90–5.

23. Cutolo M, Sulli A, Smith V. Assessing microvascular changes in systemic sclerosis diagnosis and management. Nat Rev Rheumatol 2010;6:578–87.

24. Mourad JJ, Priollet P, Girerd X, et al. The wall to lumen ratio of the radial artery in patients with Raynaud's phenomenon. J Vasc Res 1997;34:298–305.

25. Rodnan GP, Myerowitz RL, Justh GO. Morphologic changes in the digital arteries of patients with progressive systemic sclerosis (scleroderma) and Raynaud phenomenon. Medicine (Baltimore) 1980;59:393–408.

26. Pauling JD, O'Donnell VB, Mchugh NJ. The contribution of platelets to the pathogenesis of Raynaud's phenomenon and systemic sclerosis. Platelets 2013;24: 503–15.

27. Herrick AL, Illingworth K, Blann A, et al. Von Willebrand factor, thrombomodulin, thromboxane, beta-thromboglobulin and markers of fibrinolysis in primary Raynaud's phenomenon and systemic sclerosis. Ann Rheum Dis 1996;55:122–7.

28. van Bon L, Affandi AJ, Broen J, et al. Proteome-wide analysis and CXCL4 as a biomarker in systemic sclerosis. N Engl J Med 2014;370:433–43.

29. Marasini B, Cugno M, Bassani C, et al. Tissue-type plasminogen activator and von Willebrand factor plasma levels as markers of endothelial involvement in patients with Raynaud's phenomenon. Int J Microcirc Clin Exp 1992;11:375–82.

30. Silveri F, De AR, Poggi A, et al. Relative roles of endothelial cell damage and platelet activation in primary Raynaud's phenomenon (RP) and RP secondary to systemic sclerosis. Scand J Rheumatol 2001;30:290–6.

31. Prete M, Fatone MC, Favoino E, et al. Raynaud's phenomenon: from molecular pathogenesis to therapy. Autoimmun Rev 2014;13:655–67.

32. Ferri C, Valentini G, Cozzi F, et al. Systemic sclerosis: demographic, clinical, and serologic features and survival in 1,012 Italian patients. Medicine 2002;81: 139–53.

33. Ennis H, Vail A, Wragg E, et al. A prospective study of systemic sclerosis-related digital ulcers: prevalence, location, and functional impact. Scand J Rheumatol 2013;42:483–6.

34. Khimdas S, Harding S, Bonner A, et al, Canadian Scleroderma Research Group. Associations with digital ulcers in a large cohort of systemic sclerosis: results from the Canadian Scleroderma Research Group registry. Arthritis Care Res (Hoboken) 2011;63:142–9.

35. Muangchan C, Canadian Scleroderma Research Group, Baron M, et al. The 15% rule in scleroderma: the frequency of severe organ complications in systemic sclerosis. A systematic review. J Rheumatol 2013;40:1545–56.

36. Manfredi A, Sebastiani M, Carraro V, et al. Prediction risk chart for scleroderma digital ulcers: a composite predictive model based on capillaroscopic, demographic and clinico-serological parameters. Clin Hemorheol Microcirc 2015; 59(2):133–43.

37. Denton CP, Krieg T, Guillevin L, et al, DUO Registry investigators. Demographic, clinical and antibody characteristics of patients with digital ulcers in systemic sclerosis: data from the DUO Registry. Ann Rheum Dis 2012;71:718–21.

38. Smith V, Decuman S, Sulli A, et al. Do worsening scleroderma capillaroscopic patterns predict future severe organ involvement? A pilot study. Ann Rheum Dis 2012;71:1636–9.

39. Ennis H, Moore T, Murray A, et al. Further confirmation that digital ulcers are associated with the severity of abnormality on nailfold capillaroscopy in patients with systemic sclerosis. Rheumatology (Oxford) 2014;53:376–7.

40. Mouthon L, Mestre-Stanislas C, Bérezné A, et al. Impact of digital ulcers on disability and health-related quality of life in systemic sclerosis. Ann Rheum Dis 2010;69:214–7.

41. Malcarne VL, Hansdottir I, McKinney A, et al. Medical signs and symptoms associated with disability, pain, and psychosocial adjustment in systemic sclerosis. J Rheumatol 2007;34:359–67.

42. Youssef P, Englert H, Bertouch J. Large vessel occlusive disease associated with CREST syndrome and scleroderma. Ann Rheum Dis 1993;52:464–6.

43. Taylor MH, McFadden JA, Bolster MB, et al. Ulnar artery involvement in systemic sclerosis (scleroderma). J Rheumatol 2002;29:102–6.

44. Zeng Y, Li M, Xu D, et al. Macrovascular involvement in systemic sclerosis: evidence of correlation with disease activity. Clin Exp Rheumatol 2012;30(2 Suppl 71): S76–80.

45. Ho M, Veale D, Eastmond C, et al. Macrovascular disease and systemic sclerosis. Ann Rheum Dis 2000;59:39–43.

46. Wan MC, Moore T, Hollis S, et al. Ankle brachial pressure index in systemic sclerosis: influence of disease subtype and anticentromere antibody. Rheumatology (Oxford) 2001;40:1102–5.

47. Chiang CH, Liu CJ, Huang CC, et al. Systemic sclerosis and risk of ischaemic stroke: a nationwide cohort study. Rheumatology (Oxford) 2013;52:161–5.

48. Man A, Zhu Y, Zhang Y, et al. The risk of cardiovascular disease in systemic sclerosis: a population-based cohort study. Ann Rheum Dis 2013;72: 1188–93.

49. Au K, Singh MK, Bodukam V, et al. Atherosclerosis in systemic sclerosis: a systematic review and meta-analysis. Arthritis Rheum 2011;63:2078–90.

50. Nannizzi-Alaimo L, Alves VL, Phillips DR. Inhibitory effects of glycoprotein IIb/IIIa antagonists and aspirin on the release of soluble CD40 ligand during platelet stimulation. Circulation 2003;107:1123–8.

51. Coleiro B, Marshall SE, Denton CP, et al. Treatment of Raynaud's phenomenon with the selective serotonin reuptake inhibitor fluoxetine. Rheumatology (Oxford) 2001;40:1038–43.

52. Hudson M, Lo E, Lu Y, et al, Canadian Scleroderma Research Group. Cigarette smoking in patients with systemic sclerosis. Arthritis Rheum 2011;63:230–8.

53. Echeverri D, Montes FR, Cabrera M, et al. Caffeine's vascular mechanisms of action. Int J Vasc Med 2010;2010:834060.

54. Kim BJ, Seo Y, Kim JH, et al. Effect of caffeine intake on finger cold-induced vasodilation. Wilderness Environ Med 2013;24:328–36.

55. Fraenkel L, Zhang Y, Chaisson CE, et al. The association of estrogen replacement therapy and the Raynaud phenomenon in postmenopausal women. Ann Intern Med 1998;129:208–11.

56. Lekakis J, Mavrikakis M, Papamichael C, et al. Short-term estrogen administration improves endothelial function in women with systemic sclerosis and Raynaud's phenomenon. Am Heart J 1998;136:905–12.

57. Lekakis J, Papamichael C, Mavrikakis M, et al. Effect of long-term estrogen therapy on brachial arterial endothelium-dependent vasodilation in women with Raynaud's phenomenon secondary to systemic sclerosis. Am J Cardiol 1998;82:1555–7, A8.

58. Eid AH, Maiti K, Mitra S, et al. Estrogen increases smooth muscle expression of alpha2C-adrenoceptors and cold-induced constriction of cutaneous arteries. Am J Physiol Heart Circ Physiol 2007;293:H1955–61.

59. Muir AH, Robb R, McLaren M, et al. The use of Ginkgo biloba in Raynaud's disease: a double-blind placebo-controlled trial. Vasc Med 2002;7:265–7.

60. Malenfant D, Catton M, Pope JE. The efficacy of complementary and alternative medicine in the treatment of Raynaud's phenomenon: a literature review and meta-analysis. Rheumatology (Oxford) 2009;48:791–5.

61. Cho SG, Go HY, Park JS, et al. Herbal prescription, DSGOST, prevents cold-induced RhoA activation and endothelin-1 production in endothelial cells. Evid Based Complement Alternat Med 2014;2014:549307.

62. Thompson AE, Shea B, Welch V, et al. Calcium-channel blockers for Raynaud's phenomenon in systemic sclerosis. Arthritis Rheum 2001;44:1841–7.

63. Vignaux O, Allanore Y, Meune C, et al. Evaluation of the effect of nifedipine upon myocardial perfusion and contractility using cardiac magnetic resonance imaging and tissue Doppler echocardiography in systemic sclerosis. Ann Rheum Dis 2005;64:1268–73.

64. Belch JJ, Newman P, Drury JK, et al. Intermittent epoprostenol (prostacyclin) infusion in patients with Raynaud's syndrome. A double-blind controlled trial. Lancet 1983;1:313–5.

65. Pope J, Fenlon D, Thompson A, et al. Iloprost and cisaprost for Raynaud's phenomenon in progressive systemic sclerosis. Cochrane Database Syst Rev 2000;(2):CD000953.

66. Roustit M, Blaise S, Allanore Y, et al. Phosphodiesterase-5 inhibitors for the treatment of secondary Raynaud's phenomenon: systematic review and meta-analysis of randomised trials. Ann Rheum Dis 2013;72:1696–9.

67. Stone AV, Koman LA, Callahan MF, et al. The effect of botulinum neurotoxin-A on blood flow in rats: a potential mechanism for treatment of Raynaud phenomenon. J Hand Surg Am 2012;37:795–802.

68. Fregene A, Ditmars D, Siddiqui A. Botulinum toxin type A: a treatment option for digital ischemia in patients with Raynaud's phenomenon. J Hand Surg Am 2009; 34:446–52.

69. Van Beek AL, Lim PK, Gear AJ, et al. Management of vasospastic disorders with botulinum toxin A. Plast Reconstr Surg 2007;119:217–26.

70. Neumeister MW. Botulinum toxin type A in the treatment of Raynaud's phenomenon. J Hand Surg Am 2010;35:2085–92.

71. Neumeister MW, Chambers CB, Herron MS, et al. Botox therapy for ischemic digits. Plast Reconstr Surg 2009;124:191–201.

72. Giuggioli D, Manfredi A, Colaci M, et al. Scleroderma digital ulcers complicated by infection with fecal pathogens. Arthritis Care Res (Hoboken) 2012;64:295–7.

73. Giuggioli D, Manfredi A, Colaci M, et al. Osteomyelitis complicating scleroderma digital ulcers. Clin Rheumatol 2013;32:623–7.

74. Korn JH, Mayes M, Matucci Cerinic M, et al. Digital ulcers in systemic sclerosis: prevention by treatment with bosentan, an oral endothelin receptor antagonist. Arthritis Rheum 2004;50:3985–93.

75. Matucci-Cerinic M, Denton CP, Furst DE, et al. Bosentan treatment of digital ulcers related to systemic sclerosis: results from the RAPIDS-2 randomised, double-blind, placebo-controlled trial. Ann Rheum Dis 2011;70:32–8.

76. Parisi S, Peroni CL, Laganà A, et al. Efficacy of ambrisentan in the treatment of digital ulcers in patients with systemic sclerosis: a preliminary study. Rheumatology (Oxford) 2013;52:1142–4.

77. Chung L, Ball K, Yaqub A, et al. Effect of the endothelin type A-selective endothelin receptor antagonist ambrisentan on digital ulcers in patients with systemic sclerosis: results of a prospective pilot study. J Am Acad Dermatol 2014;71: 400–1.

78. Abou-Raya A, Abou-Raya S, Helmii M. Statins: potentially useful in therapy of systemic sclerosis-related Raynaud's phenomenon and digital ulcers. J Rheumatol 2008;35:1801–8.

79. Kuwana M, Kaburaki J, Okazaki Y, et al. Increase in circulating endothelial precursors by atorvastatin in patients with systemic sclerosis. Arthritis Rheum 2006;54:1946–51.

80. Kuwana M, Okazaki Y, Kaburaki J. Long-term beneficial effects of statins on vascular manifestations in patients with systemic sclerosis. Mod Rheumatol 2009;19:530–5.

81. Rehberger P, Beckheinrich-Mrowka P, Haustein UF, et al. Prostacyclin analogue iloprost influences endothelial cell-associated soluble adhesion molecules and growth factors in patients with systemic sclerosis: a time course study of serum concentrations. Acta Derm Venereol 2009;89:245–9.

82. Ghofrani HA, D'Armini AM, Grimminger F, et al, CHEST-1 Study Group. Riociguat for the treatment of pulmonary arterial hypertension. N Engl J Med 2013;369: 319–29.

83. Nihtyanova SI, Brough GM, Black CM, et al. Clinical burden of digital vasculopathy in limited and diffuse cutaneous systemic sclerosis. Ann Rheum Dis 2008;67: 120–3.

84. Zulian F, Corona F, Gerloni V, et al. Safety and efficacy of iloprost for the treatment of ischaemic digits in paediatric connective tissue diseases. Rheumatology (Oxford) 2004;43:229–33.

85. Kotsis SV, Chung KC. A systematic review of the outcomes of digital sympathectomy for treatment of chronic digital ischemia. J Rheumatol 2003;30:1788–92.

Management of Systemic-Sclerosis-Associated Interstitial Lung Disease

Katherine Culp Silver, MD[a], Richard M. Silver, MD[b],*

KEYWORDS

- Interstitial lung disease (ILD) • Systemic sclerosis (SSc) • Cyclophosphamide
- Rituximab • Stem cell transplant

KEY POINTS

- Interstitial lung disease (ILD) is the leading cause of mortality for patients with SSc.
- Early diagnosis is critical for managing patients with scleroderma-associated interstitial lung disease (SSc-ILD).
- Pulmonary function tests (PFTs) and high-resolution computed tomographic (HRCT) chest imaging are used for screening and management.
- Immunosuppression can be beneficial, but better therapies are needed.

INTRODUCTION

In the past 35 years, since the introduction of angiotensin-converting enzyme inhibitor therapy as the first effective treatment of scleroderma renal crisis, SSc-ILD has become the leading SSc-related cause of death.[1] In the largest study to date, SSc-ILD accounted for 35% of all disease-related deaths.[2] Thus the management of patients with SSc-ILD is of paramount importance. This article presents a brief discussion of the current knowledge of the pathogenesis of SSc-ILD, because such research may ultimately lead to targeted and more effective management of SSc-ILD. This article then discusses the current state of management of SSc-ILD, beginning with early detection, followed by a discussion of disease staging and risk stratification, and finally a review of current and future treatment options.

The authors have nothing to disclose.
[a] Adult & Pediatric Rheumatology, Medical University of South Carolina, Suite 816, Clinical Sciences Building, 96 Jonathan Lucas Street, Charleston, SC 29425, USA; [b] Division of Rheumatology & Immunology, Medical University of South Carolina, Suite 816, Clinical Sciences Building, 96 Jonathan Lucas Street, Charleston, SC 29425, USA
* Corresponding author.
E-mail address: silverr@musc.edu

PATHOGENESIS OF SSC-ILD

Despite several decades of intense investigation, the pathogenesis of SSc-ILD remains unclear. It is likely that SSc-ILD represents a complex interplay between innate and acquired immunity, inflammation, and fibrosis, but the exact sequence of events remains uncertain. As lung biopsy is seldom required to establish a diagnosis of SSc-ILD, insight into the pathogenesis of SSc-ILD has been hampered by a relative lack of access to lung tissue, particularly early in the course of the disease when the greatest insight on disease initiation and mechanisms might be gained. When biopsy is performed, the SSc lung histopathology typically shows interstitial fibrosis with temporal homogeneity and with only a modest inflammatory cell infiltrate (ie, fibrotic nonspecific interstitial pneumonia [NSIP]).[3] Cellular NSIP and usual interstitial pneumonia (UIP) are seen in a smaller proportion of cases.

Recent studies looking at gene expression profiles provide molecular insights into the pathogenesis of SSc-ILD (**Table 1**). Although not completely concordant, lung tissue gene expression and bronchoalveolar lavage (BAL) studies of early- and late-stage SSc-ILD demonstrate abnormal expression of markers of macrophage migration and activation, as well as upregulated expression of transforming growth factor (TGF)-β and interferon-regulated genes.[4–6] Genome-wide association studies have found the gene for chemokine (C-X-C motif) ligand 4 (CXCL4), among others, to be highly and differentially expressed in certain patients with SSc, and a recent proteome-wide analysis found serum levels of CXCL4 to be correlated with lung fibrosis.[7] Polymorphisms at loci for additional genes have also been reported to be associated with the presence and/or severity of pulmonary fibrosis (see **Table 1**).[3,8] Such genetic and molecular insights will likely lead to the future development of predictive serum biomarkers, as well as the development of safe and targeted therapies for patients with SSc-ILD.[3,9]

CLINICAL MANIFESTATIONS

Pulmonary involvement is common, occurring in over 80% of patients with SSc, and is often a significant source of morbidity and mortality.[10] Lung involvement can occur in all subsets of the disease including limited cutaneous SSc, diffuse cutaneous SSc, and SSc sine scleroderma, and it can affect all aspects of the respiratory tract including the parenchyma, vasculature, airways, pleura, and musculature.[11]

Table 1
Gene expression and associations with SSc-ILD

Proposed Biologic Function	Associations with SSc-ILD
Alveolar epithelial homeostasis	SP-B, HGF
Immune regulation	IRAK-1, IRF-5, NLRP1, CXCL4, OAS1, IFI44, CCL18, CD163
Fibroblast activation/matrix remodeling	COL1A, CTGF, MMP-12

Abbreviations: CCL18, chemokine [C-C motif] ligand 18; CD163, cluster of differentiation 163; COL1A, collagen, type I, alpha I; CTGF, CCN2 or connective tissue growth factor; CXCL4, chemokine [C-X-C motif] ligand 4; HGF, hepatocyte growth factor; IFI44, interferon-induced protein 44; IRAK-1, interleukin-1 receptor-associated kinase 1; IRF5, interferon regulatory factor 5; MMP-12, matrix metalloproteinase 12; NLRP1, NACHT, LRR, and PYD domains-containing protein 1; OAS1, 2′,5′-oligoadenylate synthetase 1; SP-B, surfactant protein B.
Adapted from Herzog EL, Mathur A, Tager AM, et al. Interstitial lung disease associated with systemic sclerosis and idiopathic pulmonary fibrosis. How similar and distinct? Arthritis Rheumatol 2014;66:1973; with permission.

Therefore, when a patient with SSc presents with symptoms of dyspnea, the differential diagnosis can be quite broad (**Box 1**).

Inflammation or fibrosis of the pulmonary interstitium, ILD, is the most frequent pulmonary manifestation in SSc. About 40% of patients have restrictive changes on PFTs while over 90% have evidence of ILD at autopsy.[12] The most common presenting symptom is dyspnea on exertion. Other indicators of ILD may include nonproductive cough, fatigue, and chest pain. The most common finding on physical examination is the presence of dry (velcrolike) crackles at the lung bases. However, some patients with SSc-ILD may not have any symptoms, and physical examination may give normal results. Therefore, the clinician must remain ever vigilant, screening all patients initially and monitoring them frequently throughout the course of their disease.

PFTs play a major role in the investigation of lung involvement in SSc (**Fig. 1**).[13] Because changes in pulmonary function can occur before the onset of significant clinical symptoms, all patients should have screening PFTs at the time of presentation. These tests should include spirometry and single-breath diffusion capacity for carbon monoxide (DL_{CO}) at a minimum. Patients with SSc-ILD have a restrictive pattern on PFTs, marked by a decreased forced vital capacity (FVC). The forced expiratory volume in the first second of expiration (FEV_1)/FVC ratio is typically normal, or sometimes even elevated, because the FEV_1 decreases in proportion to the decline in FVC. In

---

Box 1
Differential diagnosis of dyspnea in SSc

1. Interstitial lung disease
2. Pulmonary vascular disease
   - Pulmonary arterial hypertension
   - Thromboembolic disease
   - Pulmonary capillary hemangiomatosis
   - Pulmonary venoocclusive disease
3. Pleural effusion
4. Spontaneous pneumothorax
5. Recurrent aspiration
6. Airways disease
   - Airflow limitation
   - Bronchiolitis obliterans
   - Follicular bronchiolitis
   - Bronchiectasis
7. Drug-associated pneumonitis
8. Lung cancer
9. Infection
10. Respiratory muscle weakness
11. Extrinsic chest wall restriction because of skin tightness
12. Anemia
13. Deconditioning

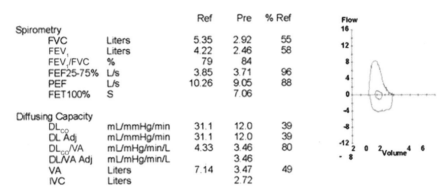

Age: 44   Gender: Male
Weight(lb): 232   Weight(kg): 105.5
Height(in): 71
Height(cm): 180 Race: Caucasian

		Ref	Pre	% Ref
Spirometry				
FVC	Liters	5.35	2.92	55
FEV₁	Liters	4.22	2.46	58
FEV₁/FVC	%	79	84	
FEF25-75%	L/s	3.85	3.71	96
PEF	L/s	10.26	9.05	88
FET100%	S		7.06	
Diffusing Capacity				
DL_CO	mL/mmHg/min	31.1	12.0	39
DL Adj	mL/mmHg/min	31.1	12.0	39
DL_CO/VA	mL/mmHg/min/L	4.33	3.46	80
DL/VA Adj	mL/mmHg/min/L		3.46	
VA	Liters	7.14	3.47	49
IVC	Liters		2.72	

Fig. 1. PFTs from a patient with SSc-ILD demonstrating a restrictive pattern on the flow volume loop, decreased FVC, and decreased DL_{CO}, but a preserved FEV₁/FVC ratio. FEV₁, forced expiratory volume in the first second of expiration.

addition, the parenchymal inflammation and fibrosis that occur in ILD lead to thickening of the interstitium, which results in a decreased DL_{CO}.[11] Thus, FVC and DL_{CO} prove to be the most important and most commonly used diagnostic markers in SSc-ILD.[13] In patients with SSc-ILD, progression of disease often varies and can be difficult to predict.[11] Therefore, monitoring these patients with serial PFTs is a crucial aspect of the management of SSc-ILD because it can provide objective evidence of improvement or deterioration of lung function.[13] In general, with serial PFTs, changes of 10% in FVC and of 15% in DL_{CO} are regarded as significant.[13]

HRCT scanning in which lung sections 3 mm or less in dimension are obtained is the most commonly used imaging modality for the evaluation of SSc-ILD (**Fig. 2**), although computed tomography with a limited number of slices to reduce radiation exposure and

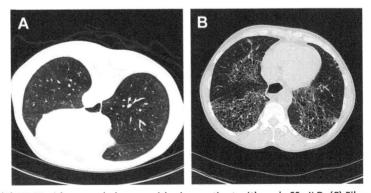

Fig. 2. (A) HRCT with ground glass opacities in a patient with early SSc-ILD. (B) Fibrosis, honeycombing, and traction bronchiectasis in a patient with more advanced disease. (*Courtesy of* J. Ravenel, MD, Charleston, SC.)

B-scale ultrasonographic imaging are being explored. The advantages of HRCT over chest radiographs include earlier detection of ILD as well as more accurate quantification of the extent of disease.[11] The most common histopathologic pattern seen in SSc-ILD is NSIP; this appears on HRCT as ground glass opacities and pulmonary fibrosis, the distribution of which is typically peripheral, bilateral, and predominantly at the lung bases. Ground glass opacities are areas of increased lung attenuation thought to represent areas of active inflammation or early fibrosis; established pulmonary fibrosis is represented by reticular thickening of the interstitium with traction bronchiectasis.[11] The extent of pulmonary fibrosis on HRCT correlates negatively with both FVC and DL_{CO}.[11] Therefore, HRCT imaging and PFTs, when used in combination, can be a powerful tool for predicting disease progression and mortality in SSc-ILD.

RISK FACTORS FOR THE PRESENCE AND PROGRESSION OF SSC-ILD

Although sensitive screening techniques identify lung disease in most patients, many cases of SSc-ILD are mild and not life threatening. Optimal management and prognosis for individual patients as well as risk stratification for future clinical trials will depend on the identification of certain clinical, serologic, radiographic, molecular, and genetic factors that individually or collectively impart a significantly increased risk for the development or progression of SSc-ILD. While useful SSc-ILD biomarkers are yet to be discovered and validated, there are several known aspects of the disease that may provide prognostic and risk information to guide monitoring and treatment:

- Gender and race: Females are at higher overall risk for developing SSc, but males are more likely to develop severe SSc-ILD. African American ethnicity is associated with earlier onset and greater severity of disease, especially SSc-ILD.[14,15]
- Extent of skin involvement: The prevalence of SSc-ILD is higher in patients with diffuse cutaneous SSc (~50%) than in those with limited cutaneous SSc (~35%).[16]
- Autoantibodies: Anti-topoisomerase I (anti-Scl-70) antibodies are strongly linked to the development SSc-ILD, with over 85% of patients with SSc who test positive for Scl-70 antibody developing pulmonary fibrosis.[17] Conversely, the presence of anti-centromere antibody seems to be associated with a much lower likelihood of development of SSc-ILD. U1-RNP, U3-RNP, Th/To, and PM/Scl autoantibodies are also associated with SSc-ILD.
- PFTs: The greatest risk of progression of SSc-ILD seems to be early in the course of disease (first 5 years). An abnormal FVC early in the disease course has been shown to be an important predictor for eventual end-stage lung disease.[18] Mortality is even more closely linked to lower values of initial PFTs (FVC and DL_{CO}) than to lung histopathology (NSIP vs UIP).[19]
- HRCT chest imaging: Patients with more extensive fibrosis on HRCT chest scans (ie, abnormalities involving >20% of the lung volume) are at significantly higher risk for rapid decline in lung function and death, compared with patients whose HRCT shows lesser involvement (<20% of the lung volume).[20] In the Scleroderma Lung Study I (SLS I), the extent of fibrosis on baseline HRCT was a useful predictor of lung disease progression when untreated and of a favorable response to treatment with cyclophosphamide compared with placebo.[21]
- Gastroesophageal reflux disease (GERD): Although cause and effect remains to be proven, an association exists between gastroesophageal reflux and ILD. The extent of SSc-ILD as assessed by PFTs and by chest HRCT is correlated with the degree of esophageal reflux.[22,23]

- Selected biomarkers: Two lung-associated glycoproteins (Krebs von den Lungen-6 and surfactant protein D) and a chemokine secreted predominantly by alveolar macrophages (C-C motif chemokine ligand 18) reflect active lung injury and may predict the progression of SSc-ILD.[24–26] Other potential plasma biomarkers include CXCL4, interleukin-6 (IL-6), chitinase 1, tenascin-C, lysyl oxidase, and IL-33.[7,27–29]

Development and validation of a composite index, composed of 2 or more of these features, is needed and helps to optimize management of individual patients as well as to provide risk stratification for future clinical trials.

TREATING SSC-ILD
Whom and When to Treat

Identifying patients at risk for the development and progression of SSc-ILD should be the first step in management. As noted above, certain demographic, clinical, serologic, and radiographic elements may identify patients at high risk who, therefore, would warrant treatment. Biomarkers and genetic markers of lung fibrosis risk will surely be developed as the era of personalized medicine emerges and as we learn more about the pathogenesis of SSc-ILD. As the initial PFTs and the extent of fibrosis on HRCT scans seem to be important determinants of outcome, Goh and colleagues[20] have proposed a simple staging system whereby extensive disease (>20% HRCT involvement) would warrant immunosuppressive treatment, whereas limited disease (<20% HRCT involvement) would not. In situations in which the extent of fibrosis on HRCT scan is indeterminate, the FVC (% predicted) would drive the decision to treat (<70% predicted) or not to treat (>70% predicted) (**Fig. 3**).[20] Another schema sets forth different criteria in determining whom to treat (**Box 2**).[30]

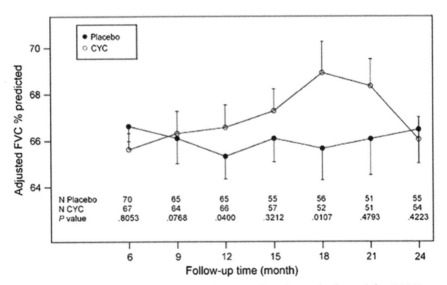

Fig. 3. Time course from 6 to 24 months of mean values (±standard error) for FVC % predicted of participants in the placebo (P) and cyclophosphamide (CYC) SLS I treatment groups. (*From* Tashkin DP, Elashoff R, Clements PJ, et al. Effects of 1-year treatment with cyclophosphamide on outcomes at 2 years in scleroderma lung disease. Am J Respir Crit Care Med 2007;176:1029, Copyright © 2015 American Thoracic Society; with permission.)

Box 2
When to initiate treatment

- Patients with limited or diffuse cutaneous SSc with dyspnea *and*
- Within 5 to 7 years after onset of signs or symptoms attributable to SSc associated with:
  - Decline in their FVC% predicted by greater than 10% in the preceding 3 to 12 months *and/or*
  - FVC % predicted of less than 70% at the time of presentation *and/or*
  - Moderate extent of ILD on baseline HRCT (defined as >20% lung involvement)[30]

How to Treat

Immunosuppression

Cyclophosphamide Over the past 25 years, immunosuppressive therapy has emerged as a treatment strategy in patients with SSc-ILD. Other forms of ILD, for example, idiopathic pulmonary fibrosis (IPF), are not as responsive to immunosuppression. Cyclophosphamide is the only such therapy thus far tested in a randomized controlled trial (RCT) and shown to be effective in treating SSc-ILD. Based on several uncontrolled and retrospective studies, the SLS I was designed as a multicenter, double-blind placebo-controlled RCT to evaluate the efficacy and safety of cyclophosphamide administered orally for 1 year in patients with symptomatic SSc-ILD and with evidence of disease activity by BAL findings and/or chest HRCT. SLS I was the first RCT to demonstrate efficacy of cyclophosphamide in improving lung function, relative to placebo, following 1 year of treatment.[21] In addition to a modest improvement in the primary end point (2.53% adjusted FVC % predicted, $P<.03$), 1 year of cyclophosphamide treatment was also associated with significant improvement in several secondary end points, for example, total lung capacity (TLC % predicted), modified Rodnan skin score (mRSS), the patient-reported outcome of dyspnea (transition dyspnea index), and several quality of life measures. After completion of 12 months of treatment with cyclophosphamide, the treatment effect on FVC % predicted increased further by 18 months, but was lost by 24 months.[31] Follow-up HRCT scans at the end of the 12-month treatment period revealed that the change in extent of fibrosis from baseline was significantly worse in the placebo group than in the cyclophosphamide treatment group ($P = .012$) and that the difference in the 12-month change in fibrosis between the 2 treatment groups significantly correlated with the favorable effect of cyclophosphamide on FVC, TLC, and dyspnea.[32]

A retrospective, multivariate regression analysis of SLS I found the maximal severity of reticular infiltrates on chest HRCT, the mRSS, and the Mahler baseline dyspnea index at baseline to be independently correlated with treatment outcomes.[33] When patients are stratified post hoc on the basis of whether 50% or more of any lung zone was involved by reticular infiltrates and/or whether patients had an mRSS of at least 23, a subgroup of patients emerges in whom the average treatment effect of cyclophosphamide on FVC was 9.81% at the 18-month assessment (ie, 6 months after completing cyclophosphamide therapy). Conversely, there was no treatment effect in patients with less-severe fibrosis on chest HRCT and a lower mRSS at baseline. This important retrospective analysis has implications for future clinical trial design in order to select patients likely to demonstrate responsiveness to the therapy to be tested.

In another trial, the Fibrosing Alveolitis in Scleroderma Trial (FAST), 45 patients with SSc-ILD were randomized to receive either intravenous cyclophosphamide

(600 mg/m^2 monthly) for 6 months followed by daily oral azathioprine 2.5 mg/kg/d (maximum 200 mg/d) or placebo infusions followed by oral placebo.[34] At 12 months, a modest but nonstatistically significant improvement in FVC was seen in the actively treated group ($P = .08$).

Based on expert consensus and evidence derived from both the SLS I and FAST trials, the european league against rheumatism (EULAR) Scleroderma Trials and Research (EUSTAR) group recommends cyclophosphamide for the treatment of SSc-ILD.[35] A recent survey of SSc experts, however, revealed a lack of consensus on treatment decisions for both induction as well as maintenance therapy.[36]

Not all patients respond to cyclophosphamide, with up to one-third of some cases showing continued decline in lung function.[37] In view of cyclophosphamide's limited efficacy, as well as short- and long-term risk of toxicity, it is clear that alternate forms of immunosuppression are needed.

Mycophenolate mofetil Mycophenolate mofetil (MMF) is regarded as a safer, less-toxic alternative to cyclophosphamide for the treatment of several immune-mediated conditions. Several uncontrolled, prospective or retrospective case series (summarized in **Table 2**)[38–49] suggest that MMF may be effective in stabilizing or, in some cases, improving lung function in patients with SSc-ILD. Based on the results of such preliminary studies, SLS II was designed to evaluate the efficacy and safety of MMF (up to 1.5 g twice daily) for 2 years when compared with oral cyclophosphamide (up to 2 mg/kg daily) for 1 year, followed by placebo for an additional year in patients with symptomatic SSc-ILD with any evidence of ground glass opacification on chest HRCT (www.clinicaltrials.gov). SLS II has completed enrollment, and release of the first year data is anticipated for 2015.

Azathioprine Published experience on the use of azathioprine for patients with SSc-ILD has been less robust and less enthusiastic than for cyclophosphamide or MMF. In a nonblinded trial comparing azathioprine with cyclophosphamide in patients with diffuse cutaneous SSc, azathioprine did not seem to halt the deterioration of lung function.[50] Azathioprine was used as maintenance therapy after monthly pulse intravenous cyclophosphamide in the FAST study, but the effect of azathioprine on the outcome of the trial is impossible to discern.[34]

Rituximab Rituximab, a monoclonal antibody directed against the B-cell CD20 antigen, has been proposed as a potential therapy for patients with SSc-ILD. In one study, rituximab therapy (n = 8) was associated with statistically significant improvement in FVC and DL$_{CO}$ and stabilization of HRCT chest imaging compared with a matched control group (n = 6) on a variety of different background medications.[51] The EUSTAR group recently evaluated rituximab treatment in a nested case-control designed study.[52] Among the 63 patients treated with rituximab, there were 9 who had SSc-ILD (defined by an FVC <70% predicted and evidence of ILD on chest HRCT). At a median follow-up of 6 months (range, 4–12 months), FVC remained stable and DL$_{CO}$ improved compared with baseline. In comparison, matched control patients with SSc-ILD showed a decline in FVC resulting in significant differences between rituximab-treated and matched controls. There was no significant difference in change in DL$_{CO}$ between rituximab-treated and matched control patients. These investigators also observed a statistically significant improvement in skin thickness (mRSS) for the rituximab-treated patients (n = 63).[52] The side effect profile of the drug seemed acceptable, and no serious adverse events were reported. Such studies support the need for a prospective, double-blind RCT to assess the efficacy and safety of rituximab in patients with SSc-ILD, either as induction or as maintenance therapy.

Autologous hematopoietic stem cell transplant Cell-based therapies, usually autologous hematopoietic stem cell transplant (HSCT), have been designed to reset an autoreactive immune system and ameliorate SSc. After high-dose cyclophosphamide and anti–thymocyte globulin with/without total body irradiation, autologous CD34$^+$ stem cells are reinfused to rescue the ablated immune system. Treatment-related mortality can be quite high because of infection and other complications, so autologous HSCT remains experimental and is offered mainly to selected patients considered to be at high risk for disease-related morbidity and mortality. Proper patient selection continues to evolve as more is learned about risk factors for treatment-related mortality.

Early success of small phase 1 and phase 2 clinical trials of autologous HSCT for patients with SSc, together with improvement in treatment-related mortality as centers gain more experience with patient selection, conditioning regimens, and supportive care, led to the conception of 2 phase 2/3 multicenter trials comparing autologous HSCT to monthly ($\times$12) intravenous cyclophosphamide, one in Europe (Autologous Stem cell Transplantation International Scleroderma [ASTIS]) and one in the United States (Scleroderma: Cyclophosphamide or Transplantation [SCOT]) (**Table 3**). Each trial has competed enrollment and patients are being followed up to compare the safety and efficacy of HSCT with the control arm of monthly pulse intravenous cyclophosphamide. Initial results of the ASTIS trial were recently published.[53] Among the 156 patients in the ASTIS trial, lung involvement was frequent (86.5% overall): chest HRCT scans gave abnormal results in 83.3% and PFTs were consistent with mild to moderate restrictive lung disease (FVC, 81.4% [18.4]; TLC, 80.7% [16.6]; DL$_{CO}$ 58.5% [14.1], each value being represented as mean [standard deviation]). Low DL$_{CO}$ may have been due to SSc-pulmonary arterial hypertension (PAH) in some cases (diagnosed in 6.6%) of the overall ASTIS study population. Follow-up of event-free survival of the intention-to-treat populations was 5.8 years at the time of the initial report. Overall, results indicate that patients treated with autologous HSCT experienced more events in the first year but had improved long-term event-free survival compared with patients treated with cyclophosphamide. During year 1, there were 11 deaths (13.9%, including 8 treatment-related deaths) in the HSCT group versus 7 deaths (9.1%, none being treatment related) in the cyclophosphamide group (risk ratio, 1.53; 95% confidence interval, 0.4–5.4). After year 2 of follow-up, there were 12 deaths (15.2%) in the HSCT group versus 13 (16.9%) in the cyclophosphamide group; after 4 years of follow-up, there were 13 deaths (16.5%) in the HSCT group versus 20 (20.6%) in the cyclophosphamide group. As expected, the mRSS decreased in both treatment groups, with a significantly greater reduction in the group receiving HSCT (mean difference, −11.1; range, −7.3 to −15.0; P<.001). There was also a statistically significant difference favoring HSCT in lung function: mean change in FVC (6.3% predicted vs −2.8% predicted) and TLC (5.1% predicted vs −1.3% predicted). No statistically significant difference in DL$_{CO}$ was observed. It is noteworthy that 7 of 8 treatment-related deaths occurred in current or former smokers; this is an important observation that should be taken into account for future trial designs of HSCT. The SCOT trial completed enrollment, and results are not expected until 2016. The Scleroderma Treatment with Autologous Transplant (STAT) trial, which is still enrolling subjects, is a multicenter, noncomparative study that will look at event-free survival when maintenance MMF therapy for up to 2 years is used after autologous HSCT.

A single-center, open-label phase 2 trial of autologous HSCT without CD34$^+$ cell selection (Autologous Stem Cell Systemic Sclerosis Immune Suppression Trial [ASSIST]) showed short-term superiority of HSCT in 10 patients who had significant regression of skin thickness (mRSS) and improvement in lung function, as well as reduction in the

Table 2
Outcomes of clinical trials of MMF for SSc

Author, Ref, Year	Patients (n)	Baseline PFTs	Regimen	Pulmonary Results
Swigris et al,[38] 2006	28 patients with CTD, 11 with SSc-ILD	FVC 65% (56%–76%)	MMF 2 g/d for median 371 d	FVC, TLC, and DL_{CO} improved by 2.3%, 4.0%, and 2.6%, respectively, which approached statistical significance
Liossis et al,[39] 2006	6 patients with SSc with ILD and alveolitis	FVC 71% (32%–80%)	MMF 2 g/d plus low-dose prednisolone for up to 12 mo	Improvement in FVC from 65.6% to 76.2% ($P = .057$) and in DL_{CO} from 64.2% to 75.4% ($P = .033$)
Nihtyanova et al,[40] 2007	172 patients with early SSc, 109 treated with MMF	Progressive ILD in 27.5% of MMF group before treatment	In MMF group, MMF for 1 y (79%) and for 12–36 mo (59%)	12% (MMF) vs 19% (control) developed progressive ILD ($P<.04$); 5-year survival 95.4% vs 85.7% ($P = .027$)
Zamora et al,[41] 2008	17 patients with SSc-ILD	FVC 72%, DL_{CO} 52%	MMF 2 g/d for 12–24 mo	At 12 mo, FVC improved by 2.6% and DL_{CO} by 1.4%. At 24 mo, FVC improved on average 2.4%
Gerbino et al,[42] 2008	13 patients with SSc-ILD with early disease	FVC 70%, DL_{CO} 51%	MMF median dose 2 g/d for median 21 mo	FVC improved by mean of 4% in contrast to a decrease of 5% during a median of 14 mo before taking MMF
Derk et al,[43] 2009	15 patients with dcSSc with disease duration ≤48 mo	FVC 99%, DL_{CO} 71.2%	MMF maximum dose 3 g/d for 13 mo	Nonsignificant trend for improvement in PFTs
Koutroumpas et al,[44] 2010	10 patients with dcSSc with ILD	FVC 79.5%, DL_{CO} 80.67%	MMF 2 g/d for median 12 mo	Significant increase in FVC and nonsignificant increase in DL_{CO} at 12 mo ($P = .04$ and .66, respectively)

Study	Population	Baseline PFTs	Treatment	Results
Le et al,[45] 2011	98 patients with dcSSc with active skin disease and mean disease duration 21.9 ± 27.6 mo	FVC 79.4%, DL_{CO} 77.4%	MMF maximum dose 3 g/d for 12 mo	Significant decrease in mRSS at 12 mo, but no significant difference in the FVC and DL_{CO}
Simeon-Aznar et al,[46] 2011	14 patients with SSc-ILD with median duration of lung symptoms of 32 mo; 10 with prior immunosuppression	FVC 64%, DL_{CO} 40%	MS 720 mg twice daily for 12 mo	Nonsignificant change in FVC or DL_{CO}; 6 patients showed >10% improvement in FVC, 5 remained stable, 3 showed >10% decline in FVC
Mendoza et al,[47] 2012	25 patients with dcSSc with disease duration <24 mo, 15 with evaluable PFTs	TLC 89.5%, DL_{CO} 69.0%	MMF mean dose 2 g/d, average duration therapy 18.2 ± 8.7 mo	Significant improvement in skin and nonsignificant change in TLC and DL_{CO}. Only 3 of 15 patients showed >10% decline in TLC
Henes et al,[48] 2013	8 evaluable patients with SSc with ILD and median disease duration 26 mo	Median FVC 78%, median DL_{CO} 75.1%	MS up to 720 mg twice daily for up to 6 mo	Stabilization of PFTs with nonsignificant changes in FVC and DL_{CO}; nonsignificant increase in lung density by HRCT histography
Panopoulos et al,[49] 2013	10 patients with SSc-ILD with mean disease duration 5.8 +/- 6.8 y	FVC 79.0%, TLC 71.5%, DL_{CO} 56.8%	MMF mean daily dose 1.5 g/d, up to >2 g/d in 8 patients, for up to 24 mo	No significant change in FVC, TLC, or DL_{CO}. Significant worsening of 2-y HRCT scores in MMF-treated patients compared with matched cyclophosphamide-treated patients

DL_{CO}, FVC, and TLC are represented as mean % predicted values.
Abbreviations: CTD, connective tissue disease; dcSSc, diffuse cutaneous systemic sclerosis; MS, mycophenolate sodium.

Table 3
Comparison of 3 randomized trials of autologous HSCT for systemic sclerosis

	ASTIS	SCOT	ASSIST
Study Design	Phase 2, nonmyeloablative, multicenter, event-free survival study	Phase 2/3, myeloablative, multicenter, event-free survival study	Phase 2, nonmyeloablative, single-center, treatment failure study
Inclusion Criteria	18–65-y-olds Disease duration ≤4 y, skin score ≥15, at least 1 predefined major organ involved or Disease duration ≤2 y, skin score ≥20, elevated acute-phase reactants, and/or proteinuria	18- to 69-y-olds Disease duration ≤5 y Diffuse cutaneous SSc, skin score ≥16 plus either pulmonary disease or prior renal crisis	18- to 60-y-olds Disease duration ≤4 y mRSS ≥15 and internal organ involvement or restricted skin involvement (mRSS ≤15) but coexistent pulmonary involvement
Exclusion criteria	Predefined severe organ damage Prior cyclophosphamide total >5 g IV or >2 mg/kg po for >3 mo	Predefined severe organ damage Prior cyclophosphamide >6 mo or >3 g/m²	Predefined severe organ damage Prior cyclophosphamide >6 mo
Mobilizing Regimen	Cyclophosphamide and G-CSF	G-CSF	Cyclophosphamide and G-CSF
Conditioning Regimen	Cyclophosphamide 200 mg/kg Rabbit ATG	Cyclophosphamide 120 mg/kg Equine ATG TBI 800 cGy (with lung and renal shielding)	Cyclophosphamide 200 mg/kg Rabbit ATG
Graft Manipulation	CD34⁺ cell selection	CD34⁺ cell selection	No CD34⁺ cell selection
Primary End Point	Survival without organ failure at 3 y	Event-free survival without organ failure at 54 mo	Improvement at 12 mo defined as a decrease in mRSS (>25% for those with initial mRSS >14) or an increase in FVC >10%
Control Arm	Cyclophosphamide 750 mg/m² IV monthly × 12; crossover to HSCT not allowed	Cyclophosphamide 750 mg/m² IV monthly × 12; crossover to HSCT not allowed	Cyclophosphamide 1000 mg/m² IV monthly × 6
Current Status	Completed; 156 patients enrolled and randomized Primary analysis reported in 2014[53]	Completed enrollment in 2011 Results pending follow-up	Completed; 19 patients enrolled and randomized (10 HSCT, 9 cyclophosphamide of whom 7 crossed over to HSCT after cyclophosphamide failure). Primary analysis reported in 2011[54] ASSIST IIb currently underway to test less-intensive conditioning regimen (clinicaltrials.gov/ct2/show/NCT01445821)

Abbreviations: ASSIST, Autologous Stem Cell Systemic Sclerosis Immune Suppression Trial; ATG, anti-thymocyte globulin; G-CSF, granulocyte colony-stimulating

extent of lung disease on chest HRCT.[54] Of the 9 control patients (cyclophosphamide-treated), 8 showed disease progression, and 7 of these patients then crossed over to HSCT therapy. After 2 years of follow-up, 11 of 18 patients showed persistent improvement in skin score, chest HRCT, and FVC (but not TLC or DL_{CO}).

Another clinical trial, STAT, is currently enrolling patients (clinicaltrials.gov/ct2/show/NCT01413100). In this clinical trial, selected patients with active SSc-ILD who have failed conventional immunosuppressive therapy will receive autologous $CD34^+$ stem cells followed by maintenance therapy with MMF for up to 2 years.

Other investigational immunosuppressive agents In addition to the aforementioned immunosuppressive treatments (**Table 4**), several other drugs with immunosuppressive properties are currently under investigation to treat SSc, including an IL-6 receptor blocker (tocilizumab), a T-cell costimulatory blocker (abatacept), and a monoclonal antibody directed against B-cell activating factor (belimumab). It remains to be seen if any of such agents will prove to be an effective therapy for SSc-ILD.

Antifibrotic therapy

Given the magnitude of the impact of fibrosis, estimated to contribute to as much as 45% of the mortality in Western developed countries,[55] the pace of development of effective antifibrotic drugs has been disappointing. The bleak picture for antifibrotic therapy to treat SSc may be improving, as new animal models that more faithfully replicate the human disease are emerging, more promising biomarkers are being developed, and greater knowledge on the mechanisms and pathways of fibrosis is being gained.[27] In 2014, the Food and Drug Administration approved 2 new drugs, pirfenidone and nintedanib, for the treatment of patients with IPF. Both drugs, which

Table 4
Summary of immunosuppressive therapies in SSc-ILD

Drug	Proposed Mechanism of Action	Status of Investigation
Cyclophosphamide	Alkylating agent that prevents cell division by cross-linking DNA strands and decreasing DNA synthesis	SLS I: multicenter, double-blind placebo-controlled RCT FAST: multicenter, double-blind placebo-controlled RCT
MMF	Exhibits a cytostatic effect on T and B lymphocytes through the inhibition of de novo guanosine nucleotide synthesis	SLS II: multicenter, double-blind placebo-controlled RCT (ongoing)
Azathioprine	Imidazolyl derivative of mercaptopurine that incorporates its metabolites into replicating DNA and halts replication	Single unblinded RCT of 60 patients
Rituximab	Monoclonal antibody directed against the CD20 antigen on B lymphocytes	Small RCT of 14 patients Nested case-control designed study
Autologous HSCT	Administration of hematopoietic progenitor cells derived from the individual with the disorder to reset an autoreactive immune system	ASTIS: phase 2, multicenter, event-free survival study SCOT: phase 2/3, multicenter, event-free survival study (ongoing) ASSIST: single-center, open-label phase 2 trial

act by downregulating the expression or signaling by TGF-β, are now undergoing preliminary safety and efficacy studies in patients with SSc-ILD. Many other new therapeutics that target specific growth factors, cytokines, or pathways (eg, monoclonal CCN2 or connective tissue growth factor antibodies, tocilizumab, endostatin-1-derived peptide, caveolin scaffolding domain), as well as multiple existing drugs that might be repurposed to treat fibrosis (eg, peroxisome proliferator-activated receptor-γ agonists [eg, rosiglitazone],[56–58] statins [rosuvastatin],[59] fluoroquinolone antibiotics [eg, ciprofloxacin],[60] and thrombin inhibitors [eg, dabigatran][61]) loom on the horizon. Given that the pathogenic mechanisms of fibrotic diseases in general and SSc in particular consist of complex networks of multiple and often redundant pathways, blocking a single molecule or pathway will likely not be sufficient and, like cancer, it may be necessary to treat patients with multiple drugs that affect different pathways.[62]

Adjunctive therapy

General measures In addition to immunosuppressive therapies, patients with SSc-ILD should receive the same supportive care measures used in other types of ILD. These measures should include supplemental oxygen (if indicated), appropriate vaccinations, and pulmonary rehabilitation therapy. Patients with SSc-ILD should receive yearly influenza vaccination and periodic vaccination against pneumococcal pneumonia. Furthermore, those patients on cyclophosphamide should receive prophylaxis against *Pneumocystis jirovecii* (formerly *Pneumocystis carinii*). In addition, the association between GERD and ILD demands aggressive management of reflux symptoms in patients with SSc. This management can be accomplished through the use of pharmacologic agents, such as proton pump inhibitors (PPIs) and H2 blockers, and augmented by nonpharmacologic methods, such as elevating the head of the bed and avoiding lying down for several hours after a meal. These general measures are not to be overlooked because they can have a significant impact on easing the symptom burden and improving the quality of life in patients with SSc-ILD (**Box 3**).

Intravenous immunoglobulin Intravenous immunoglobulin (IV Ig) therapy has been shown to be useful as adjunctive therapy in some patients with myositis-associated ILD not responding to steroids and immunosuppressive drugs.[63] When SSc is

---

Box 3
Supportive care measures

- Supplemental oxygen
  - If indicated
- Appropriate vaccinations
  - Influenza
  - *Streptococcus pneumoniae*
- Prophylaxis against *Pneumocystis jirovecii*
  - If indicated
- Pulmonary rehabilitation
- Treatment of GERD
  - Medications (PPI, H2 antagonists)
  - Reflux precautions

complicated by an inflammatory myositis, ILD occurs not infrequently (eg, anti-PM/Scl-antibody-positive patients). In such cases, IV Ig therapy might be a useful adjunctive measure when conventional treatment proves inadequate.

Lung transplant Given the lack of highly effective medical therapy, some patients with SSc progress to end-stage lung disease. Lung transplant should be considered for selected patients in whom the condition progresses despite medical therapy, but transplant centers have been reluctant to consider patients with SSc-ILD given the high prevalence of gastroesophageal reflux and its attendant risks for aspiration, bronchiolitis obliterans, and allograft rejection. Querying the United Network for Organ Sharing database revealed that less than 1% (196 of 25,260) of all lung transplants performed in the United States from January 1988 to January 2013 for end-stage lung disease were done in patients with SSc.[64] Nevertheless, reviews of transplant outcomes comparing patients with SSc with those with IPF and with PAH have shown similar 2-year and 5-year outcomes for patients with SSc (72% and 55%, respectively).[65,66] A recent review of the medical literature reporting outcomes of lung transplant in patients with SSc found no reports of recurrence of SSc in the lung allograft.[67] In a recent report of 10 patients with SSc, severity of GERD was shown to impact the 1-year survival rate.[68] Esophageal pH monitoring should be considered in patients with SSc-ILD, because this test could identify those patients in whom laparoscopic antireflux surgery should be performed to minimize GERD and its detrimental effects while awaiting lung transplant.

REFERENCES

1. Steen VD, Medsger TA Jr. Changes in causes of death in systemic sclerosis. Ann Rheum Dis 2007;66:940–4.
2. Tyndal AJ, Banert B, Vonk M, et al. Causes and risk factors for death in systemic sclerosis: a study from the EULAR Scleroderma Trials and Research (EUSTAR) database. Ann Rheum Dis 2010;69:1809–15.
3. Herzog EL, Mathur A, Tager AM, et al. Interstitial lung disease associated with systemic sclerosis and idiopathic pulmonary fibrosis. How similar and distinct? Arthritis Rheum 2014;66:1967–78.
4. Hsu E, Shi H, Jordan RM, et al. Lung tissues in patients with systemic sclerosis have gene expression patterns unique to pulmonary fibrosis and pulmonary hypertension. Arthritis Rheum 2011;63:783–94.
5. Christmann RB, Sampaio-Barros P, Stifano G, et al. Association of interferon- and transforming growth factor-β–regulated genes and macrophage activation with systemic sclerosis–related progressive lung fibrosis. Arthritis Rheum 2014;66:714–25.
6. Lindahl GE, Stock CJ, Shi-Wen X, et al. Microarray profiling reveals suppressed interferon stimulated gene program in fibroblasts from scleroderma-associated interstitial lung disease. Respir Res 2013;14:80.
7. van Bon L, Affandi AJ, Broen J, et al. Proteome-wide analysis and CXCL4 as a biomarker in systemic sclerosis. N Engl J Med 2014;370:433–43.
8. Assassi S, Radstake TR, Mayes MD, et al. Genetics of scleroderma: implications for personalized medicine? BMC Med 2013;11:9.
9. Silver RM, Feghali-Bostwick C. Molecular insights into systemic sclerosis-associated interstitial lung disease. Arthritis Rheum 2014;66:485–7.
10. Ferri C, Valentini G, Cozzi F, et al. Systemic sclerosis: demographic, clinical, and serologic features and survival in 1,012 Italian patients. Medicine (Baltimore) 2002;81(2):139–53.

11. Hant FN, Herpel LB, Silver RM. Pulmonary manifestations of scleroderma and mixed connective tissue disease. Clin Chest Med 2010;31(3):433–49.
12. Varga J. Systemic sclerosis: an update. Bull NYU Hosp Jt Dis 2008;66(3): 198–202.
13. Behr J, Furst DE. Pulmonary function tests. Rheumatology (Oxford) 2008; 47(Suppl 5):v65–7.
14. Silver RM, Bogatkevich G, Tourkina E, et al. Racial differences between blacks and whites with systemic sclerosis. Curr Opin Rheumatol 2012;24(6):642–8.
15. Steen V, Domsic RT, Lucas M, et al. A clinical and serologic comparison of African American and Caucasian patients with systemic sclerosis. Arthritis Rheum 2012; 64:2986–94.
16. Walker UA, Tyndall A, Czirják L, et al. Clinical risk assessment of organ manifestations in systemic sclerosis: a report from the EULAR Scleroderma Trials and Research Group database. Ann Rheum Dis 2007;66:754–63.
17. Briggs DC, Vaughan RW, Welsh KI, et al. Immunogenetic prediction of pulmonary fibrosis in systemic sclerosis. Lancet 1991;338(8768):661–2.
18. Morgan C, Knight C, Lunt M, et al. Predictors of end stage lung disease in a cohort of patients with scleroderma. Ann Rheum Dis 2003;62:146–50.
19. Bouros D, Wells AU, Nicholson AG, et al. Histopathologic subsets of fibrosing alveolitis in patients with systemic sclerosis and their relationship to outcome. Am J Respir Crit Care Med 2002;165:1581–6.
20. Goh NS, Desai SR, Veeraraghavan S, et al. Interstitial lung disease in systemic sclerosis: a simple staging system. Am J Respir Crit Care Med 2008;177:1248–54.
21. Tashkin D, Elashoff R, Clements P, et al. Cyclophosphamide versus placebo in scleroderma lung disease. N Engl J Med 2006;25(354):2655–66.
22. Savarino E, Bazzica M, Zentilin P, et al. Gastroesophageal reflux and pulmonary fibrosis in scleroderma: a study using pH-impedance monitoring. Am J Respir Crit Care Med 2009;179:408–13.
23. Christmann RB, Wells AU, Capelozzi VL, et al. Gastroesophageal reflux incites interstitial lung disease in systemic sclerosis: clinical, radiologic, histopathologic, and treatment evidence. Semin Arthritis Rheum 2010;40(3):241–9.
24. Hant FN, Ludwicka-Bradley A, Wang HJ, et al, Scleroderma Lung Study Research Group. Surfactant protein D and KL-6 as serum biomarkers of interstitial lung disease in patients with scleroderma. J Rheumatol 2009;36:773–80.
25. Yanaba K, Hasegawa M, Hamaguchi Y, et al. Longitudinal analysis of serum KL-6 levels in patients with systemic sclerosis: association with the activity of pulmonary fibrosis. Clin Exp Rheumatol 2003;21:429–36.
26. Kodera M, Hasegawa M, Komura K, et al. Serum pulmonary and activation-regulated chemokine/CCL18 levels in patients with systemic sclerosis. Arthritis Rheum 2005;52:2889–96.
27. Fan MH, Feghali-Bostwick CA, Silver RM. Update on scleroderma-associated interstitial lung disease. Curr Opin Rheumatol 2014;26:630–6.
28. De Laurentis A, Sestini P, Pantelidis P, et al. Serum interleukin-6 is predictive of early functional decline and mortality in interstitial lung disease associated with systemic sclerosis. J Rheumatol 2013;40:435–46.
29. Lee CG, Herzog EL, Ahangari F, et al. Chitinase 1 is a biomarker for and therapeutic target in scleroderma-associated interstitial lung disease that augments TGF-β signaling. J Immunol 2012;189:2635–44.
30. Au K, Khanna D, Clements PJ, et al. Current concepts in disease-modifying therapy for systemic sclerosis-associated interstitial lung disease: lessons from clinical trials. Curr Rheumatol Rep 2009;11:111–9.

31. Tashkin DP, Elashoff R, Clements PJ, et al. Effects of 1-year treatment with cyclo-phosphamide on outcomes at 2 years in scleroderma lung disease. Am J Respir Crit Care Med 2007;176:1026–34.

32. Goldin JG, Lynch DA, Strollo DC, et al. Follow-up HRCT after treatment of scleroderma-interstitial lung disease with cyclophosphamide demonstrates evidence for treatment effect. Am J Respir Crit Care Med 2008;177(A768):91.

33. Roth MD, Tseng CH, Clements PJ, et al. Predicting treatment outcomes and responder subsets in scleroderma-related interstitial lung disease. Arthritis Rheum 2011;63(9):2797–808.

34. Hoyles RK, Ellis RW, Wellsbury J, et al. A multicenter, prospective, randomized, double-blind, placebo-controlled trial of corticosteroids and intravenous cyclo-phosphamide followed by oral azathioprine for the treatment of pulmonary fibrosis in scleroderma. Arthritis Rheum 2006;54:3962–70.

35. Kowal-Bielecka O, Landewe R, Avouac J, et al. EULAR recommendations for the treatment of systemic sclerosis: a report from the EULAR Scleroderma Trials and Research group (EUSTAR). Ann Rheum Dis 2009;60:620–8.

36. Walker KM, Pope J, Participating members of the Scleroderma Clinical Trials Consortium (SCTC), Canadian Scleroderma Research Group (CSRG). Treatment of systemic sclerosis complications: what to use when first-line treatment fails–a consensus of systemic sclerosis experts. Semin Arthritis Rheum 2012;42:42–55.

37. Mittoo S, Wigley FM, Wise RA, et al. Long term effects of cyclophosphamide treatment on lung function and survival in scleroderma patients with interstitial lung disease. Open Rheumatol J 2011;5:1–6.

38. Swigris JJ, Olson AL, Fischer A, et al. Mycophenolate mofetil is safe, well tolerated, and preserves lung function in patients with connective tissue disease-related interstitial lung disease. Chest 2006;130:30–6.

39. Liossis SN, Bounas A, Andonopoulos AP. Mycophenolate mofetil as first-line treatment improves clinically evident early scleroderma lung disease. Rheumatology (Oxford) 2006;45:1005–8.

40. Nihtyanova SI, Brough GM, Black CM, et al. Mycophenolate mofetil in diffuse cutaneous systemic sclerosis – a retrospective analysis. Rheumatology (Oxford) 2007;46:442–5.

41. Zamora AC, Wolters PJ, Collard HR, et al. Use of mycophenolate mofetil to treat scleroderma-associated interstitial lung disease. Respir Med 2008;102:150–5.

42. Gerbino AJ, Goss CH, Molitor JA. Effect of mycophenolate mofetil on pulmonary function in scleroderma-associated interstitial lung disease. Chest 2008;133:455–60.

43. Derk CT, Grace E, Shenin M, et al. A prospective open-label study of mycophenolate mofetil for the treatment of diffuse systemic sclerosis. Rheumatology 2009;48:1595–9.

44. Koutroumpas A, Ziogas A, Alexiou I, et al. Mycophenolate mofetil in systemic sclerosis-associated interstitial lung disease. Clin Rheumatol 2010;29:1167–8.

45. Le EN, Wigley FM, Shah AA, et al. Long-term experience of mycophenolate mofetil for treatment of diffuse cutaneous systemic sclerosis. Ann Rheum Dis 2011;70:1104–7.

46. Simeon-Aznar CP, Fonollosa-Pia V, Tolosa-Vilella C, et al. Effect of mycophenolate sodium in scleroderma-related interstitial lung disease. Clin Rheumatol 2011;30:1393–8.

47. Mendoza FA, Nagle SJ, Lee JB, et al. A prospective observational study of mycophenolate mofetil treatment in progressive diffuse cutaneous systemic sclerosis of recent onset. J Rheumatol 2012;39:1241–7.

48. Henes JC, Horger M, Amberger C, et al. Enteric-coated mycophenolate sodium for progressive systemic sclerosis – a prospective open-label study with CT histography for monitoring pulmonary fibrosis. Clin Rheumatol 2013; 32:673–8.

49. Panopoulos ST, Bournia VK, Trakada G, et al. Mycophenolate versus cyclophosphamide for progressive interstitial lung disease associated with systemic sclerosis: a 2-year case control study. Lung 2013;191:483–9.

50. Nadashkevich O, Davis P, Fritzler M, et al. A randomized unblinded trial of cyclophosphamide versus azathioprine in the treatment of systemic sclerosis. Clin Rheumatol 2006;25:205–12.

51. Daoussis D, Liossis SN, Tsamandas AC, et al. Experience with rituximab in scleroderma: results from a 1-year, proof-of-principle study. Rheumatology (Oxford) 2010;49:271–80.

52. Jordan S, Distler JH, Maurer B, et al, On behalf of the EUSTAR rituximab study group. Effects and safety of rituximab in systemic sclerosis: an analysis from the European Scleroderma Trial and Research (EUSTAR) group. Ann Rheum Dis 2014. http://dx.doi.org/10.1136/annrheumdis-2013-204522.

53. Van Laar JM, Farge D, Sont JK, et al, EBMT/EULAR Scleroderma Study Group. Autologous hematopoietic stem cell transplantation vs intravenous pulse cyclophosphamide in diffuse cutaneous systemic sclerosis. A randomized clinical trial. JAMA 2014;311:2490–8.

54. Burt RK, Shah SJ, Dill K, et al. Autologous non-myeloablative haemopoietic stem-cell transplantation compared with pulse cyclophosphamide once per month for systemic sclerosis (ASSIST): an open-label, randomized phase 2 trial. Lancet 2011;378:498–506.

55. Wynn TA. Common and unique mechanisms regulate fibrosis in various fibroproliferative diseases. J Clin Invest 2007;117:524–9.

56. Antonelli A, Ferri C, Ferrari SM, et al. Peroxisome proliferator-activated receptor γ agonists reduce cell proliferation and viability and increase apoptosis in systemic sclerosis fibroblasts. Br J Dermatol 2013;168(1):129–35.

57. Bogatkevich GS, Highland KB, Akter T, et al. The PPARγ agonist rosiglitazone is antifibrotic for scleroderma lung fibroblasts: mechanisms of action and differential racial effects. Pulm Med 2012;2012:545172.

58. Wei J, Ghosh AK, Sargent JL, et al. PPARγ downregulation by TGFβ in fibroblast and impaired expression and function in systemic sclerosis: a novel mechanism for progressive fibrogenesis. PLoS One 2010;5(11):e13778.

59. Timár O, Szekanecz Z, Kerekes G, et al. Rosuvastatin improves impaired endothelial function, lowers high sensitivity CRP, complement and immuncomplex production in patients with systemic sclerosis–a prospective case-series study. Arthritis Res Ther 2013;15:R105.

60. Ruben EC, Manuel VR, Agustin OR, et al. Ciprofloxacin utility as antifibrotic in the skin of patients with scleroderma. J Dermatol 2010;37:323–9.

61. Atanelishvili I, Liang J, Akter T, et al. Thrombin increases lung fibroblast survival while promoting alveolar epithelial cell apoptosis via the endoplasmic reticulum stress marker, CCAAT enhancer-binding homologous protein. Am J Respir Cell Mol Biol 2014;50:893–902.

62. Rosenbloom J, Mendoza FA, Jimenez SA. Strategies for anti-fibrotic therapies. Biochim Biophys Acta 2013;1832:1088–103.

63. Suzuki Y, Hayakawa H, Miwa S, et al. Intravenous immunoglobulin therapy for refractory interstitial lung disease associated with polymyositis/dermatomyositis. Lung 2009;187(3):201–6.

64. De Cruz S, Ross D. Lung transplantation in patients with scleroderma. Curr Opin Rheumatol 2013;25:714–8.
65. Shitrit D, Amitai A, Peled N, et al. Lung transplantation in patients with scleroderma: case series, review of the literature, and criteria for transplantation. Clin Transplant 2009;23:178–83.
66. Schachna L, Medsger TA Jr, Dauber JH, et al. Lung transplantation in scleroderma compared with idiopathic pulmonary fibrosis and idiopathic pulmonary arterial hypertension. Arthritis Rheum 2006;54:3954–61.
67. Khan IY, Singer LG, de Perrot M, et al. Survival after lung transplantation in systemic sclerosis. A systematic review. Respir Med 2013;107:2081–7.
68. Fisichella PM, Reder NP, Gagermeier J, et al. Usefulness of pH monitoring in predicting the survival status of patients with scleroderma awaiting lung transplantation. J Surg Res 2014;189:232–7.

Systemic Sclerosis

Gastrointestinal Disease and Its Management

Genevieve Gyger, MD*, Murray Baron, MD

KEYWORDS

- Systemic sclerosis • Gastroesophageal reflux • Dysmotility • Gastroparesis
- Pseudo-obstruction • Constipation • Fecal incontinence • Esophagus

KEY POINTS

- A multidisciplinary approach with a gastroenterologist, nutritionist, and often a speech therapist is mandatory in all patients with severe gastrointestinal involvement.
- Oral cavity abnormalities are common in systemic sclerosis and can be severe.
- Gastroesophageal reflux may trigger or worsen interstitial lung disease.
- All patients with scleroderma should be screened for malnutrition.
- Treatment of fecal incontinence starts with optimization of the constipation treatment.
- Probiotics may be useful in patients with bloating and distension and small intestinal bacterial overgrowth.
- Well-powered prospective studies are needed to determine the effect of immunosuppressive treatment on the onset of gastrointestinal tract disease, especially in early systemic sclerosis.

INTRODUCTION

The gastrointestinal (GI) tract is the most frequently involved internal organ in systemic sclerosis (SSc), affecting more than 90% of patients.[1] The most frequent GI involvement is the esophagus, followed by the ano-rectum and small bowel, but any part of the GI tract can be affected, from the mouth to the anus.

This article reviews the pathophysiology of GI tract involvement in SSc and discusses the investigations and management of the disease. **Table 1** shows the most commonly used investigations to assess the GI tract in SSc, and treatments are listed in **Table 2**.

The authors have no relevant financial disclosures to make.
Division of Rheumatology, Jewish General Hospital, McGill University, Suite A725, 3755 Cote St Catherine Road, Montreal, Quebec H3T 1E2, Canada
* Corresponding author.
E-mail address: genevieve.gyger@mcgill.ca

Table 1
Common investigation for gastrointestinal involvement in SSC

Organ	Abnormality	Investigations
Esophagus	Esophagitis, stricture, Barrett esophagus	EGD
	Dysmotility, GER	Esophageal transit (nuclear medicine)
	Stricture, dysmotility	Barium swallow
	Dysmotility	Manometry
Stomach	Dysmotility	Gastric emptying study (nuclear medicine)
	GAVE, gastritis, ulcers, adenocarcinoma	EGD
Small bowel	Pseudo-obstruction	Plain abdominal radiography and CT scan
	Pneumatosis intestinalis and perforation	
	SIBO	Lactulose and glucose
	—	Hydrogen breath test
Colon	Dilatation, volvulus, perforation	Plain radiography and CT scan
	Large wide mouth diverticula	—
	Telangiectasis	Colonoscopy
Anorectum	Incontinence	Anorectal manometry
	—	Endosonography
	—	Defecography

PATHOPHYSIOLOGY OVERVIEW

Sjogren[2] has proposed an interesting hypothesis of the pathophysiology of the GI tract in SSc that includes 4 stages: vasculopathy, neural dysfunction, smooth muscle atrophy, and tissue fibrosis.[2] The earliest lesion may be vascular with mild changes in intestinal

Table 2
Treatment options

Organ	Problem	Treatment
Oral cavity	Dry mouth	Artificial saliva, sugar free gum and candies
		Secretagogues pilocarpine, cevimeline
Esophagus	GER	Lifestyle changes
		Proton-pump inhibitors
		H2 receptor antagonist
		Sucralfate
		Antacid
	Dysmotility	Prokinetic agents: Domperidone
		Cisapride
Small bowel	Small intestinal bacterial overgrowth	Antibiotics, probiotics
	Pseudo-obstruction	Treat SIBO, domperidone, metoclopramide
		Octreotide $\pm$ erythromycin, cisapride
	Pneumatosis intestinalis	Antibiotics, nasal oxygen or elementary diet or parenteral nutrition
Colon	Constipation	Diet rich in fiber, stool softener, polyethylene glycol, Probiotics, possibly prucalopride
Anorectum	Fecal incontinence	Treat constipation, sphincter muscle training
		Sacral nerve stimulation

permeability, transport, and absorption. This stage is followed by neural dysfunction, in which the patient starts to have clinical symptoms such as dysphagia, gastroesophageal reflux (GER), and bloating. At that phase, prokinetic drugs may largely reverse the functional abnormalities. The vasculopathy and neural dysfunction then lead to the third stage of smooth muscle atrophy. This stage is marked by only partial response to drugs. Finally, the end stage is muscle fibrosis, when drugs are no longer useful.

Recent detection of circulating autoantibodies to myenteric neurons in a substantial number of SSc patients suggests an autoimmune etiology of the neural dysfunction in the GI tract.[3,4] The muscarinic 3 receptor (M3R) is the principal receptor of acetylcholine, which is the main excitatory neurotransmitter regulating GI tract motility. Antibodies to the M3R receptor have been found in SSc and may inhibit this excitatory effect of acetylcholine and cause dysmotility.[3–5] Intravenous infusion of immunoglobulin could neutralize SSc antibodies against M3R, and this was suggested in a recent study.[5]

ORAL CAVITY

Oral cavity abnormalities are common in SSc and can be severe but are frequently disregarded. SSc patients have significantly more missing teeth and periodontal disease, less saliva production, and a smaller interincisal distance compared with controls.[6] The number of missing teeth is associated with worse hand function, the presence of GER, and decreased saliva production.[7] Oral health-related quality of life of SSc patients is significantly impaired and is not captured well by physician assessment of disease severity.[8] Use of adaptive devices such as flossers, powered oscillating-rotating toothbrushes, and orofacial exercise to improve oral health should be considered.

ESOPHAGUS

The esophagus is the most common internal organ involvement in SSc, affecting 70% to 90% of the patients. The distal two-thirds of the esophagus is affected, with smooth muscle atrophy, fibrosis, and dilatation. There is a weakened lower esophageal sphincter with profound loss of peristaltic action and dysmotility.[1] A dilated esophagus on a computed tomography (CT) of the chest is common in SSc.[9] As many as 50% of patients will be completely asymptomatic. Investigations with esophagealgastroduodenoscopy (EGD) in 13 patients with early SSc without GI tract symptoms found reflux esophagitis in 77% of patients, dysmotility of the distal esophagus in 85%, gastritis in 95% (31% erosive gastritis) and *Helicobacter pylori* in 38% of the patients.[10] Some pathologic conditions of the upper GI tract were found in all the patients.

Symptoms of esophageal dysfunction range from asymptomatic to dysphagia, GER, nausea, or vomiting with poor eating and severe weight loss.[1] Damage from GER includes peptic esophagitis that can progress to erosive esophagitis, bleeding, and frank ulceration if untreated. Peptic stricture, fistulae, and an achalasialike syndrome may also occur as well as candida esophagitis owing to poor emptying of the esophagus and immunosuppressive treatment. Barrett's esophagus with ultimate adenocarcinoma is also increased in SSc patients.[11] Moreover, GER is suggested to be a risk factor for the development of interstitial lung disease (ILD).[12]

Diagnosis of Esophageal Involvement

Diagnosis of dysmotility is made with esophageal manometry, barium swallow, or esophageal transit (scintigraphy). Other possible tests used include impedance monitoring.[13] Although manometry is the gold standard, it is an invasive test and is not convenient. A study on the comparison of esophageal scintigraphy with manometry showed that esophageal scintigraphy is nearly as accurate as manometry in detecting esophageal hypomotility.[14] It can also detect GER. In contrast, barium contrast studies lack sensitivity and specificity, and interpretation is largely subjective, but it gives qualitative information about structure (eg, diverticula, strictures, masses). Esophageal transit is, therefore, a good examination to assess esophageal involvement. However, if there is any doubt about the results on clinical grounds, one should pursue the investigation with manometry. They are no clear recommendations, however, concerning what test should be used, and choice depends largely on the center where the tests are performed.

EGD allows evaluation of ulcers, esophagitis, stricture, Barret's disease, and adenocarcinoma.

Treatment of Esophageal Involvement

First-line management of symptomatic esophageal involvement implies lifestyle changes such as smoking cessation, eating smaller portions more often, eating the last meal of the day earlier, and elevation of the head of the bed. Dietary interventions include modifying the texture of food, such as purees or scrambled eggs. Yogurt may be recommended and avoidance of exacerbating food groups, such as spicy food. Despite the lack of specific randomized, controlled trials, some experts feel that all SSc patients should be treated with proton-pump inhibitor (PPI), for the prevention of GER, GER-related ILD, esophageal ulcers, and strictures.[15] Some patients require twice-daily PPI administration with addition of H2 blockers at night. Sucralfate, a sucrose sulfate-aluminium complex that binds to the mucosa, thus creating a physical barrier that impairs diffusion of hydrochloric acid in the gastrointestinal tract and prevents degradation of mucus by acid, may also be added as a cytoprotector. Although there may be concern that suppression of gastric acid could alter the bacterial flora of the upper gastrointestinal tract and lead to complications such as cancer and enteric or other infections and malabsorption, the current evidence indicates that this suppression rarely leads to clinical disease.[16] Because it is suggested that GER may be responsible for some of the interstitial lung disease in SSc, it may be especially important to prevent GER although it is not yet clear if gastric acid or other components of gastric juices might be responsible for lung damage.[17–19] The use of PPI in patients with idiopathic ILD showed a stabilization of the disease in a case series of 4 patients followed up for 3 to 6 years.[20] Moreover, in a prospective study of 6 SSc patients with ILD possibly attributed to GER, intensive treatment with antireflux therapy showed stability of their lung disease after 1 year.[21] More studies are needed to assess the role of aggressive dysmotility treatment and prevention of ILD in SSc.

Treatment of symptomatic esophageal dysmotility, such as dysphagia and severe GER not well controlled on PPI, includes prokinetic drugs. Cisapride, a serotonin 5-HT$_4$ receptor agonist, was found to have a beneficial effect on gastric emptying and lowering esophageal pressure in a small, randomized, controlled study.[22] However, because of concerns about long QT syndrome and severe arrhythmias, the medication was withdrawn from the market in some countries. Domperidone, a dopamine D2 receptor antagonist, increases the tonus of the inferior esophagus and the peristalsis of the antrum and is a safer drug than cisapride. Domperidone can be used in patients with dysphagia. A dose of 10 to 20 mg up to 4 times a day 30 minutes before meals can be tried. However, the risk of sudden death and severe arrhythmia has been a recent concern and may be increased in patients taking doses higher than 30 mg/d or in patients older than 60 years. It should be used with caution in patients with heart failure or arrhythmia and if used concomitantly with another QT-prolonging drugs. Because it is usually helpful in SSc patients, a reasonable approach is to monitor the QT with electrocardiogram when the dose is increased.

Strictures are most often treated with dilatation via endoscopic balloon dilatators or bougies. Barrett esophagus can be treated by radiofrequency ablation, endoscopic thermal therapy, photodynamic therapy, cryotherapy, or endoscopic mucosal resection.[23]

STOMACH

Gastric dysfunction has been reported in up to 50% of patients, and manifestations include early satiety, bloating, nausea, and abdominal discomfort. However, it is not rare to have normal gastric function with severe esophageal and small bowel dysmotility. Patients with gastroparesis symptoms must be referred to a gastroenterologist to rule out gastric outlet obstruction. Gastric dysfunction also increases severity of GER.[1] Normally, liquids distribute throughout the stomach and empty after a pressure gradient from the proximal stomach to the duodenum. Solids, in contrast, are pushed toward the antrum by smooth muscle contraction. Reduced frequency of the slow waves by the gastric pacemaker (bradygastria), which initiates contraction to crush food against a closed pylorus, combined with decreased muscle activity and increased compliance in the fundus, can result in significant dysfunction.[24] Assessment of delayed emptying is done with gastric emptying studies in nuclear medicine, but a motility capsule can also be used as well as gastric emptying breath test, antroduodenal manometry, and electrogastrography.[13]

Treatment to increase gastric motility includes prokinetic drugs such as metoclopramide, domperidone, erythromycin, and cisapride.[13,24,25] Metoclopramide, a central and peripheral dopamine receptor antagonist, has been found to augment antral, duodenal, and jejuna motor activity.[24] A dose of 10 to 15 mg 4 times a day is the maximum dose. However, concern about long-term use and extrapyramidal side effects limits its use. A long-term dose of 10 mg hs (every night at bed time) is reasonable if symptoms persist despite domperidone and erythromycin. Domperidone, (10–20 mg daily, up to 4 times a day) does not cross the brain barrier and is therefore safer. Erythromycin at low dose (100–150 mg daily, up to 4 times a day) imitates the effect of motilin on the gastrointestinal motility and acts directly on smooth muscle. One must be careful about the combination of domperidone and erythromycin, as both increase QT. Mosapride, a selective $5-HT_4$ agonist, has been found to accelerate gastric emptying but was not studied in SSc.[15]

Iron deficiency or, less commonly, severe bleeding, can occur secondary to gastric vascular ectasia (GAVE), know as *watermelon stomach*.[1] In one study, the prevalence was 5.6%, and it was more prevalent in early diffuse cutaneous SSc and late-onset limited SSc.[26] A second in early severe diffuse SSc found a prevalence of 22.3%.[27] Anemia is present in most patients affected by GAVE. Histologic studies show mucosal capillary dilatations containing fibrin thrombi, fibromuscular hyperplasia, and reactive foveal epithelial changes.[28] GAVE has also been recently linked to the presence of anti-RNA pol III antibodies and renal crisis and the absence of antitopoisomerase I antibodies.[27,29] Patients with chronic gastrointestinal bleeding can be treated with laser or argon plasma coagulation.

EGD can evaluate isolated telangiectasis or GAVE and gastric ulcer. Capsule endoscopy can also be used.

SMALL BOWEL

Patients with small bowel involvement have alterations of peristalsis, which can lead to stasis of the intestinal contents with small intestine bacterial overgrowth (SIBO). This can lead to bloating, abdominal discomfort, steatorrhea, and diarrhea. More severe cases can present with pseudo-obstruction, pneumatosis intestinalis, malabsorption, weight loss, and ultimately malnutrition, although some patients remain asymptomatic.

Small Intestine Bacterial Overgrowth

SIBO is common in SSc, affecting 33% to 43% of the patients.[30] Microorganisms increase in number or there is a change in the balance of the flora, which leads to competition for essential nutrients (such as vitamin B12), deconjugation of bile acids leading to fat malabsorption, reduced food intake, and diarrhea. Malabsorption has been found in 10% to 25% of patients and is a poor prognostic factor, with a 50% mortality rate at 8.5 years.[31,32] Although SIBO is the main cause of malabsorption, other causes include exchange disturbances, dysfunction of adsorptive epithelial cells, lymphatic drainage disturbance, and reduced intestinal permeability secondary to fibrosis of the mucosa and submucosa. Finally, chronic intestinal ischemia, pancreatic dysfunction, and primary biliary cirrhosis are other causes of malabsorption.[30]

Method of diagnosis of SIBO includes jejunal culture, breath tests, and Schilling tests. None of these methods has been validated, but the hydrogen breath test (often glucose or lactulose) is the most widely used and is noninvasive. However, this method is not available in all centers. Therefore, irrespective of the result of the breath test, a trial of antibiotic can be prescribed in a patient with high suspicion of SIBO. If the patient responds to the treatment, SIBO is likely.

Treatment of SIBO includes antibiotics that are usually prescribed initially for 10 or 21 days and then a 10- to 14-day course can be repeated if diarrhea recurs.[25] Patients who quickly relapse could need a 10-day course of antibiotic every month. Moreover, some patients who relapse whenever the antibiotics are discontinued need continuous treatment, with alternating antibiotics every 2 weeks. The choices of antibiotics are listed in **Table 3**.[25] For the treatment of diarrhea, opioid analogues such as loperamide can also be used but with caution to prevent pseudo-obstruction. In cases of fat malabsorption caused by SIBO, cholestyramine or other bile salt sequestrant may be helpful.

A few small studies have found very good results in patients with SIBO (not SSc patients) treated with probiotics.[33,34] One study in SSc patients complaining of bloating and distension showed significant improvement in bloating or distension after 2 months of daily probiotic use.[35] Probiotics exert various beneficial effects including strengthening the barrier function of the gut, inhibiting several pathogens, modifying

Table 3 Oral antibiotics for small intestinal bacterial overgrowth	
Agent	**Dose**
Tetracycline	250 mg qid
Doxycycline	100 mg bid
Minocycline	100 mg bid
Amoxicillin-clavulanic acid	875 mg bid
Cephalexin+	250 mg qid
Metronidazole	250 mg tid
Ciprofloxacin	500 mg bid
Norfloxacin	400 mg bid
Chloramphenicol	250 mg qid

the inflammatory response of the bowel, reducing visceral hypersensitivity, and having immunomodulatory activities.[36,37] Moreover, they are generally regarded as safe. Align (bifidobacterium infantis; Procter and Gambles, USA), Culturelle (lactobacillus; i-Health Inc, USA), or yogurt with probiotics can be used. There is no consensus regarding how and when to use probiotics, but daily use without antibiotics[35] or use after an antibiotic course has been suggested.[25,34]

Pseudo-Obstruction

In severe cases, small bowel motility disturbance can manifest by obstipation, which can progress to pseudo-obstruction.[1] Pseudo-obstruction is characterized by signs and symptoms of intestinal obstruction in the absence of an occluding lesion of the intestinal lumen (Fig. 1). An abdominal CT scan should be performed to exclude a mechanical cause. Pseudo-obstruction can be of various degrees of severity, may be either acute or chronic, and may be present in up to 40% of patients.[31] Scintigraphy, MRI and dynamic MRI are other tests that can be used to diagnose pseudo-obstruction.

Treatment of pseudo-obstruction includes promotility agents and, in severe cases, small bowel rest with nasogastric tube. Promotility agents include domperidone, metoclopramide, and erythromycin. In refractory cases, treatment with octreotide, 50 to 100 μg subcutaneously at bedtime is prescribed with good results.[38–40] Long-acting–release octreotide, 20 mg intramuscularly every month may be needed if relapse occurs and may limit the short relapses.[41] It is safer to start with a monthly intramuscular dose equivalent to the total daily dose per month and then increase slowly. Addition of erythromycin to octreotide could also be beneficial.[42] Octreotide has some disadvantages, including inhibitory effects on gastric emptying, pancreatic secretions, gallbladder contractions, and increased incidence of cholelithiasis. Surgical intervention in pseudo-obstruction is often complicated by prolonged ileus and is, therefore, discouraged.

Pneumatosis Cystoid Intestinalis

Pneumatosis cystoid intestinalis is a rare condition and a poor prognostic sign. It is characterized by air cysts in the mucosa and submucosa of the small bowel wall,

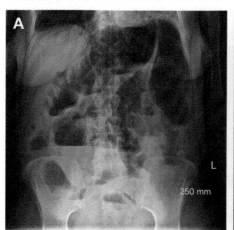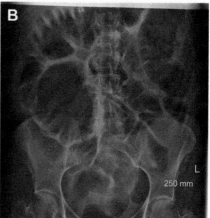

Fig. 1. Pseudo-obstruction. (*A*) There are multiple air fluid levels and dilatation of bowel in keeping with pseudo-obstruction. (*B*) Important dilatation of the colon secondary to pseudo-obstruction in scleroderma.

probably secondary to increased luminal pressure in the context of excessive gas production. It can be seen on plain radiography, but CT of the abdomen is a more sensitive test (**Fig. 2**). Pneumatosis cystoid intestinalis can present with nausea, abdominal pain, weight loss, vomiting, or diarrhea although often is asymptomatic. A picture of spontaneous benign pneumoperitoneum occurs if cysts rupture. The condition is usually sterile and is not an intra-abdominal catastrophe in which surgery is indicated. The lack of leukocytosis, fever, or rebound tenderness favors the benign etiology. Conservative treatment is mandatory, with antibiotics, nasal oxygen or elementary diet, or total parenteral nutrition.

Vascular Ectasias in the Small Intestine

Vascular ectasias in the small intestine may be the source of bleeding and can be diagnosed with capsule endoscopy or enteroscopy.[13]

Malabsorption

Malabsorption is unfortunately a common manifestation of gastrointestinal involvement and has to be recognized to prevent further deterioration with malnutrition. Malabsorption affects 10% to 25% of patients and is a poor prognostic factor, with a 50% mortality rate at 8.5 years. Patients present with diarrhea and weight loss, and it can be confirmed with the following tests: serum methylmalonic acid, zinc, 25-OH vitamin D levels, vitamin K level, or prothombin time and hydrogen breath test, as malabsorption is mainly caused by SIBO. Malabsorption can ultimately lead to malnutrition.

Malnutrition

The risk of malnutrition is high in SSc, with more than 28% of patients at medium or high risk of malnutrition in a Canadian study.[43] Experts agree that all patients with SSc should be screened for malnutrition.[25] Weight loss is the most sensitive indicator of malnutrition and should be performed at regular intervals. Experts agree that a weight loss of 1% to 2% in the previous week, greater than 5% in the previous month, greater than 7.5% in the previous 3 months, or greater than 10% in the previous year is a significant weight loss. A body mass index less than 18.5 kg/m^2 is also suggestive of protein-energy malnutrition.[25]

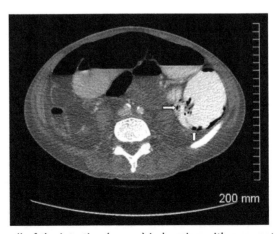

Fig. 2. Air in the wall of the intestine (*arrows*) in keeping with pneumatosis intestinalis.

Malnutrition is usually attributed to SIBO[44] or to dysmotility disorder of the GI tract leading to early satiety, nausea, and vomiting. However, malnutrition was also associated with the physician assessment of global disease severity, suggesting that malnutrition could also be secondary to causes other than GI tract involvement.[43]

An easy screening tool such as the Malnutrition Universal Screening Tool may be helpful. This tool was developed by the British Association for Parenteral and Enteral Nutrition and combines body mass index and weight measures.[25,30]

Tests should be obtained to confirm malnutrition. These tests include those performed to rule out malabsorption (previous discussion) and prealbumin (transthyretin). Albumin is not a sensitive or specific marker of protein energy malnutrition but more a negative acute phase reactant.[30]

Patients with a positive malnutrition screening result must be seen by a team including a rheumatologist, gastroenterologist, and nutritionist. A referral to a mental health worker may also be necessary if symptoms of depression are present. Referral to a speech pathologist to assess swallowing and protection of the airway should be considered as well as a consultation with a dentist.[25]

Specific treatment for all possible causes should be initiated. These include treatment of dysmotility of the esophagus, stomach, and small bowel and SIBO. In refractory cases, enteral nutrition via a jejunostomy (preferable to a gastrostomy) or parenteral nutrition must be started. Because of increased risk of infections with parenteral nutrition and vascular thrombosis and liver failure, enteral nutrition should first be tried.[25] However, some patients with severe gastric and small bowel dysmotility will not tolerate enteral nutrition.

Unusual Specific Radiologic Findings

CT scan may also show abnormalities that are specific for SSc, such as "hide-bound" small bowel, characterized by diffuse dilatation of the small bowel with closely packed valvulae conniventes, affecting more frequently the duodenum and jejunum.[45]

COLON

Colonic involvement can affect 20% to 50% of the patients.[15] Reduced colonic motility and prolonged transit cause constipation. Rectorrhagia can occur secondary to telangiectasias in the colon or rectum (watermelon rectum) causing iron deficiency anemia. Other potential complications of colonic involvement include ulcerations, perforations, stricture, volvulus, and infarct.[30] Pseudodiverticula are common, with secondary rectal prolapse.[30] Although surgery is avoided as much as possible because of fear of prolonged ileus postoperation, occasionally it is mandatory, with successful results. Colonic involvement can be evaluated with sigmoidoscopy and colonoscopy, manometry, sitz markers (opaque markers that when swallowed can be used to measure transit time in the large intestine), and radiologic imaging, such as plain radiography and CT scan.[13,14]

Treatment of constipation includes a diet rich in fiber, stool softener, and polyethylene Glycol (Lax-A-Day, Pendopharm, Canada). Osmotic laxatives can aggravate bloating and discomfort. Treatment of concomitant SIBO with antibiotics and use of probiotics can be useful. Prucalopride, a selective high-affinity $5-HT_4$ receptor agonist, is safe and useful in patients with opiod-induced constipation.[46] Preclinical studies show that prucalopride induces giant migrating contractions, stimulates proximal colonic motility, enhances gastro-pyloro-duodenal motility, and accelerates delayed gastric emptying.[46] It was also studied in patients with chronic intestinal pseudo-obstruction with good results, improving pain, nausea, vomiting, and bloating.[47]

However, only case reports are published in SSc.[48] It is a promising drug in SSc. Studies are needed before drawing recommendations. Sacral nerve stimulation in constipation is useful in chronic idiopathic constipation, but there is no study in SSc, and it is expensive.[15]

Investigations to assess colon involvement include colonoscopy, radiologic imaging, manometry, barium enema, and scintigraphy.[13]

ANORECTAL INVOLVEMENT

The anorectal involvement affects 50% to 70% of the patients. More than 20% of patients will suffer from fecal incontinence.[49] Patients can also suffer from rectal prolapse. Tenesmus and pain during defecation can also occur in SSc patients. SSc patients, regardless of their symptoms of fecal incontinence, have thin and atrophic sphincters.[49] Patients with fecal incontinence, however, had a higher anal sensory threshold compared with asymptomatic patients, suggesting a neuropathic cause to fecal incontinence.[50] Diagnostic tests include manometry, defecography, and endoscopy. Treatment of fecal incontinence starts with optimization of the constipation treatment, sphincter muscle training, and, in more severe cases, sacral nerve stimulation.[1,13,51]

Tests performed to assess anorectal involvement include anorectal manometry, sigmoidoscopy and colonoscopy, defecography, endosonography, and surface electromyography.[13]

LIVER

The most frequent associated disease is primary biliary cirrhosis (PBC).[13] PBC is associated with antimitochondrial antibodies (AMAs) in 80% to 96.5% of the cases and is also associated with CENP-B antibodies.[52] PBC occurs in 2% to 18% of SSc patients.[52] Diagnosis is suspected in patients with an elevation of alkaline phosphatase, increased immunoglobulin M levels, and positive AMAs. At least half of the patients are asymptomatic at diagnosis. The utilization of AMA (MIT3) and sp100 antibodies as a combined marker of PBC improved detection of PBC in patients with SSc.[52] Patients with suspected PBC should be referred to the gastroenterologist or hepatologist, as it is a treatable disease. It seems that PBC associated with SSc has a slower progression, with increased time to death by liver disease or time to liver transplant compared with PBC-alone patients.[53]

Subclinical elevation of transaminases can be present in the context of anti-inflammatory or analgesic use or other immunosuppressive therapy potentially affecting the liver.

PANCREAS

Although rare, pancreatic involvement in SSc has been reported and should be suspected in patients with steatorrhea not improving on antibiotics. Fat malabsorption can be investigated with a qualitative test of the stool and then confirmed by a 72-hour fecal fat collection. Treatment with specific enzymes might be needed.[13]

GASTROINTESTINAL INVOLVEMENT, DEPRESSION, AND QUALITY OF LIFE

Between 36% and 65% of patients with SSc have clinically significant symptoms of depression.[54] The number of gastrointestinal symptoms was significantly associated with depression, after controlling for sociodemographic factors and global estimates of SSc severity and duration.[55] Another study found that depression was highly and independently associated with worse functioning of the upper gastrointestinal tract.[56]

Depressed patients had worse GI scale scores and reflux and constipation scales were independently associated with worse depression score.[57]

Patients with SSc GI involvement also suffer from reduced quality of life.[58,59] A recent study from a population-based cohort of patients with SSc found that patients with lower bowel symptoms had reduced quality of life compared with the general population. Moreover, GI complaints and especially abdominal pain and bloating affects patients' social lives.[58]

IMMUNOSUPPRESSIVE THERAPY FOR GASTROINTESTINAL INVOLVEMENT

There is no evidence suggesting that immunosuppressive therapy prevents GI disease in SSc. Our own data from a longitudinal cohort study of early SSc subjects (<3 years of disease since onset of first non-Raynaud's symptom) without severe GI disease found that exposure to immunosuppressive therapy (for other disease manifestations) did not protect against the onset of severe GI disease (Canadian Scleroderma Research Group data, unpublished, 2013). Unfortunately, data from trials of immunosuppression for SSc rarely report GI outcomes and, therefore, provide little insight on this question. Well-powered prospective studies are needed to determine the effect of immunosuppressive treatment on the onset of GI tract disease, especially in early SSc.

ALTERNATIVE AND FUTURE TREATMENTS

Although studies on complementary and alternative treatments are small and scarce, modalities such as acupressure and transcutaneous electroacupuncture may improve GI functioning or symptoms in SSc patients.[60] Recent publications highlight the non-nutritional effects of food that could have a therapeutic role in chronic gastrointestinal diseases.[61] Studies on a diet low in fermentable oligosaccharides, disaccharides, monosaccharides, and polyols (FODMAPs) in patients suffering from irritable bowel syndrome (IBS) suggest a potential role of this diet in patients with this condition.[62] Given a potential role of SIBO in the pathophysiology of IBS and that ingestion of FOD-MAPs increases the delivery of readily fermentable substrates and water to the distal small intestine and colon resulting in luminal distension and gas,[62] there might be a role for this diet in SSc. Studies in SSc, however, are needed.

SUMMARY

Gastrointestinal involvement is common and appears early in SSc, and the esophagus is the first internal organ affected in most patients. We cannot rely on patients' symptoms for early diagnosis, as 50% of them are asymptomatic. Therefore, treatment of all SSc patients with a PPI to prevent GI and lung complications might be considered. Physicians must also appropriately question their patients regarding possible GI involvement and start therapy early, before irreversible damage occurs. A multidisciplinary approach with a gastroenterologist, nutritionist, and often a speech therapist is mandatory in all patients with severe GI involvement. Finally, patients with GI disease often suffer from depression and have a reduced quality of life; therefore, referral to a psychiatrist or psychologist should be considered.

REFERENCES

1. Forbes A, Marie I. Gastrointestinal complications: the most frequent internal complications of systemic sclerosis. Rheumatology (Oxford) 2009;48(Suppl 3):iii36–9.

2. Sjogren RW. Gastrointestinal features of scleroderma. Curr Opin Rheumatol 1996; 8:569–75.

3. Kawaguchi Y, Nakamura Y, Matsumoto I, et al. Muscarinic-3 acetylcholine receptor autoantibody in patients with systemic sclerosis: contribution to severe gastrointestinal tract dysmotility. Ann Rheum Dis 2009;68:710–4.

4. Singh J, Mehendiratta V, Del Galdo F, et al. Immunoglobulins from scleroderma patients inhibit the muscarinic receptor activation in internal anal sphincter smooth muscle cells. Am J Physiol Gastrointest Liver Physiol 2009;297:G1206–13.

5. Singh J, Cohen S, Mehendiratta V, et al. Effects of scleroderma antibodies and pooled human immunoglobulin on anal sphincter and colonic smooth muscle function. Gastroenterology 2012;143:1308–18.

6. Baron M, Hudson M, Tatibouet S, et al. The Canadian systemic sclerosis oral health study: orofacial manifestations and oral health-related quality of life in systemic sclerosis compared with the general population. Rheumatology (Oxford) 2014;53:1386–94.

7. Baron M, Hudson M, Tatibouet S, et al. Relationship between disease characteristics and orofacial manifestations in systemic sclerosis: Canadian Systemic Sclerosis Oral Health Study III. Arthritis Care Res (Hoboken) 2015;67:681–90.

8. Baron M, Hudson M, Tatibouet S, et al. The Canadian Systemic Sclerosis Oral Health Study II: the relationship between oral and global health-related quality of life in systemic sclerosis. Rheumatology (Oxford) 2014;54(4):692–6.

9. Vonk MC, van Die CE, Snoeren MM, et al. Oesophageal dilatation on high-resolution computed tomography scan of the lungs as a sign of scleroderma. Ann Rheum Dis 2008;67:1317–21.

10. Thonhofer R, Siegel C, Trummer M, et al. Early endoscopy in systemic sclerosis without gastrointestinal symptoms. Rheumatol Int 2012;32:165–8.

11. Wipff J, Coriat R, Masciocchi M, et al. Outcomes of Barrett's oesophagus related to systemic sclerosis: a 3-year EULAR Scleroderma Trials and Research prospective follow-up study. Rheumatology (Oxford) 2011;50:1440–4.

12. American Thoracic Society. Idiopathic pulmonary fibrosis: diagnosis and treatment. International consensus statement. American Thoracic Society (ATS), and the European Respiratory Society (ERS). Am J Respir Crit Care Med 2000; 161:646–64.

13. Kirby DF, Chatterjee S. Evaluation and management of gastrointestinal manifestations in scleroderma. Curr Opin Rheumatol 2014;26:621–9.

14. Clements PJ, Becvar R, Drosos AA, et al. Assessment of gastrointestinal involvement. Clin Exp Rheumatol 2003;21:S15–8.

15. Hansi N, Thoua N, Carulli M, et al. Consensus best practice pathway of the UK scleroderma study group: gastrointestinal manifestations of systemic sclerosis. Clin Exp Rheumatol 2014;32:S-214–21.

16. Williams C, McColl KE. Review article: proton pump inhibitors and bacterial overgrowth. Aliment Pharmacol Ther 2006;23:3–10.

17. Raghu G, Freudenberger TD, Yang S, et al. High prevalence of abnormal acid gastro-oesophageal reflux in idiopathic pulmonary fibrosis. Eur Respir J 2006; 27:136–42.

18. Tobin RW, Pope CE 2nd, Pellegrini CA, et al. Increased prevalence of gastroesophageal reflux in patients with idiopathic pulmonary fibrosis. Am J Respir Crit Care Med 1998;158:1804–8.

19. Zhang XJ, Bonner A, Hudson M, et al. Association of gastroesophageal factors and worsening of forced vital capacity in systemic sclerosis. J Rheumatol 2013;40:850–8.

20. Raghu G, Yang ST, Spada C, et al. Sole treatment of acid gastroesophageal reflux in idiopathic pulmonary fibrosis: a case series. Chest 2006;129:794–800.
21. de Souza RB, Borges CT, Capelozzi VL, et al. Centrilobular fibrosis: an underrecognized pattern in systemic sclerosis. Respiration 2009;77:389–97.
22. Kahan A, Chaussade S, Gaudric M, et al. The effect of cisapride on gastrooesophageal dysfunction in systemic sclerosis: a controlled manometric study. Br J Clin Pharmacol 1991;31:683–7.
23. Spechler SJ, Sharma P, Souza RF, et al. American Gastroenterological Association technical review on the management of Barrett's esophagus. Gastroenterology 2011;140:e18–52 [quiz: e13].
24. Butt S, Emmanuel A. Systemic sclerosis and the gut. Expert Rev Gastroenterol Hepatol 2013;7:331–9.
25. Baron M, Bernier P, Cote LF, et al. Screening and therapy for malnutrition and related gastro-intestinal disorders in systemic sclerosis: recommendations of a North American expert panel. Clin Exp Rheumatol 2010;28:S42–6.
26. Peeters TL. The potentials of erythromycin derivatives in the treatment of gastrointestinal motility disorders. Z Gesamte Inn Med 1991;46:349–54 [in German].
27. Hung EW, Mayes MD, Sharif R, et al. Gastric antral vascular ectasia and its clinical correlates in patients with early diffuse systemic sclerosis in the SCOT trial. J Rheumatol 2013;40:455–60.
28. Ingraham KM, O'Brien MS, Shenin M, et al. Gastric antral vascular ectasia in systemic sclerosis: demographics and disease predictors. J Rheumatol 2010;37: 603–7.
29. Selinger CP, Ang YS. Gastric antral vascular ectasia (GAVE): an update on clinical presentation, pathophysiology and treatment. Digestion 2008;77:131–7.
30. Gyger G, Baron M. Gastrointestinal manifestations of scleroderma: recent progress in evaluation, pathogenesis, and management. Curr Rheumatol Rep 2012;14:22–9.
31. Sjogren RW. Gastrointestinal motility disorders in scleroderma. Arthritis Rheum 1994;37:1265–82.
32. Jaovisidha K, Csuka ME, Almagro UA, et al. Severe gastrointestinal involvement in systemic sclerosis: report of five cases and review of the literature. Semin Arthritis Rheum 2005;34:689–702.
33. Soifer LO, Peralta D, Dima G, et al. Comparative clinical efficacy of a probiotic vs. an antibiotic in the treatment of patients with intestinal bacterial overgrowth and chronic abdominal functional distension: a pilot study. Acta Gastroenterol Latinoam 2010;40:323–7 [in Spanish].
34. Gabrielli M, Lauritano EC, Scarpellini E, et al. Bacillus clausii as a treatment of small intestinal bacterial overgrowth. Am J Gastroenterol 2009;104:1327–8.
35. Frech TM, Khanna D, Maranian P, et al. Probiotics for the treatment of systemic sclerosis-associated gastrointestinal bloating/distention. Clin Exp Rheumatol 2011;29:S22–5.
36. Bures J, Cyrany J, Kohoutova D, et al. Small intestinal bacterial overgrowth syndrome. World J Gastroenterol 2010;16:2978–90.
37. Urdaci MC, Bressollier P, Pinchuk I. Bacillus clausii probiotic strains: antimicrobial and immunomodulatory activities. J Clin Gastroenterol 2004;38:S86–90.
38. Perlemuter G, Cacoub P, Chaussade S, et al. Octreotide treatment of chronic intestinal pseudoobstruction secondary to connective tissue diseases. Arthritis Rheum 1999;42:1545–9.
39. Soudah HC, Hasler WL, Owyang C. Effect of octreotide on intestinal motility and bacterial overgrowth in scleroderma. N Engl J Med 1991;325:1461–7.
40. Owyang C. Octreotide in gastrointestinal motility disorders. Gut 1994;35:S11–4.

41. Descamps V, Duval X, Crickx B, et al. Global improvement of systemic sclero-derma under long-term administration of octreotide. Eur J Dermatol 1999;9:446–8.
42. Verne GN, Eaker EY, Hardy E, et al. Effect of octreotide and erythromycin on idio-pathic and scleroderma-associated intestinal pseudoobstruction. Dig Dis Sci 1995;40:1892–901.
43. Baron M, Hudson M, Steele R. Malnutrition is common in systemic sclerosis: re-sults from the Canadian scleroderma research group database. J Rheumatol 2009;36:2737–43.
44. Attar A. Digestive manifestations in systemic sclerosis. Ann Med Interne (Paris) 2002;153:260–4 [in French].
45. Pickhardt PJ. The "hide-bound" bowel sign. Radiology 1999;213:837–8.
46. Sloots CE, Rykx A, Cools M, et al. Efficacy and safety of prucalopride in patients with chronic noncancer pain suffering from opioid-induced constipation. Dig Dis Sci 2010;55:2912–21.
47. Emmanuel AV, Kamm MA, Roy AJ, et al. Randomised clinical trial: the efficacy of prucalopride in patients with chronic intestinal pseudo-obstruction–a double-blind, placebo-controlled, cross-over, multiple n = 1 study. Aliment Pharmacol Ther 2012;35:48–55.
48. Boeckxstaens GE, Bartelsman JF, Lauwers L, et al. Treatment of GI dysmotility in scleroderma with the new enterokinetic agent prucalopride. Am J Gastroenterol 2002;97:194–7.
49. Thoua NM, Schizas A, Forbes A, et al. Internal anal sphincter atrophy in patients with systemic sclerosis. Rheumatology (Oxford) 2011;50:1596–602.
50. Thoua NM, Abdel-Halim M, Forbes A, et al. Fecal incontinence in systemic scle-rosis is secondary to neuropathy. Am J Gastroenterol 2012;107:597–603.
51. Kenefick NJ, Vaizey CJ, Nicholls RJ, et al. Sacral nerve stimulation for faecal in-continence due to systemic sclerosis. Gut 2002;51:881–3.
52. Assassi S, Fritzler MJ, Arnett FC, et al. Primary biliary cirrhosis (PBC), PBC auto-antibodies, and hepatic parameter abnormalities in a large population of sys-temic sclerosis patients. J Rheumatol 2009;36:2250–6.
53. Rigamonti C, Shand LM, Feudjo M, et al. Clinical features and prognosis of primary biliary cirrhosis associated with systemic sclerosis. Gut 2006;55:388–94.
54. Thombs BD, Taillefer SS, Hudson M, et al. Depression in patients with systemic sclerosis: a systematic review of the evidence. Arthritis Rheum 2007;57:1089–97.
55. Thombs BD, Hudson M, Taillefer SS, et al. Prevalence and clinical correlates of symptoms of depression in patients with systemic sclerosis. Arthritis Rheum 2008;59:504–9.
56. Nietert PJ, Mitchell HC, Bolster MB, et al. Correlates of depression, including overall and gastrointestinal functional status, among patients with systemic scle-rosis. J Rheumatol 2005;32:51–7.
57. Bodukam V, Hays RD, Maranian P, et al. Association of gastrointestinal involve-ment and depressive symptoms in patients with systemic sclerosis. Rheuma-tology (Oxford) 2011;50:330–4.
58. Franck-Larsson K, Graf W, Ronnblom A. Lower gastrointestinal symptoms and quality of life in patients with systemic sclerosis: a population-based study. Eur J Gastroenterol Hepatol 2009;21:176–82.
59. Johnson SR, Glaman DD, Schentag CT, et al. Quality of life and functional status in systemic sclerosis compared to other rheumatic diseases. J Rheumatol 2006;33:1117–22.

60. Sallam HS, McNearney TA, Chen JD. Acupuncture-based modalities: novel alternative approaches in the treatment of gastrointestinal dysmotility in patients with systemic sclerosis. Explore (NY) 2014;10:44–52.
61. Gibson PR, Muir JG. Non-nutritional effects of food: an underutilized and understudied therapeutic tool in chronic gastrointestinal diseases. J Gastroenterol Hepatol 2013;28(Suppl 4):37–40.
62. Magge S, Lembo A. Low-FODMAP Diet for Treatment of Irritable Bowel Syndrome. Gastroenterol Hepatol 2012;8:739–45.

Scleroderma Renal Crisis

Loïc Guillevin, MD*, Luc Mouthon, MD, PhD

KEYWORDS

- Scleroderma renal crisis • Systemic sclerosis • Arterial hypertension
- Acute renal failure • Angiotensin-converting-enzyme inhibitors

KEY POINTS

- Scleroderma renal crisis is a rare complication of systemic sclerosis (SSc) that remains severe.
- Prompt recognition and initiation of therapy with an angiotensin-converting-enzyme inhibitor offer the best chance to achieve a good outcome.
- SSc prevalence is poorly known, with disparities among countries.

INTRODUCTION

Systemic sclerosis (SSc) is a connective tissue disease involving multiple organs characterized by excessive collagen deposition, autoimmunity, vascular hyperreactivity, and obliterative microvascular phenomena.[1] Vascular injury can manifest as Raynaud phenomenon, digital ischemia, pulmonary arterial hypertension, or scleroderma renal crisis (SRC).[2]

Before the late 1970s, SRC was rarely described,[3] occurring in 8.3% of one series of SSc patients,[4] and was responsible for the deaths of 10.5% in another study.[5] Interstitial lung disease and pulmonary arterial hypertension are now the 2 main causes of SSc-related deaths, with SRC developing in 5% of the patients, mainly those with diffuse cutaneous SSc (dcSSc).

Routine use of angiotensin-converting-enzyme inhibitors (ACEIs) has dramatically improved outcomes, with a 12-month decline in mortality from 76% to less than 15% in the United States.[6] Despite the improved prognosis, SRC remains a severe SSc manifestation, and functional outcome and survival remain poor: 65% at 5 years.[5–7] For the recent series, 5-year survival was 60%.[8] Herein, SRC epidemiology, main characteristics, outcomes, and treatments are reviewed.

Department of Internal Medicine, Centre de Référence Maladies Systémiques et Auto-Immunes Rares, Hôpital Cochin, Assistance Publique-Hôpitaux de Paris, Université Paris Descartes, Paris, France
* Corresponding author.
E-mail address: loic.guillevin@cch.aphp.fr

Rheum Dis Clin N Am 41 (2015) 475–488
http://dx.doi.org/10.1016/j.rdc.2015.04.008
0889-857X/15/$ – see front matter
rheumatic.theclinics.com

DEFINITION

SRC is a rare SSc manifestation that presents as new-onset accelerated hypertension or rapidly deteriorating renal function, frequently accompanied by signs of microangiopathic hemolysis.[9] Clinical symptoms comprise headaches, signs of encephalopathy, sometimes seizures, and stroke. Hypertensive retinopathy with perturbed vision and blurring is frequent. Fever, malaise, and poor general condition are usual. Some patients develop pulmonary edema because of salt and water retention, sometimes with oliguria. Myocardial involvement, pericarditis, and rhythm disturbances are associated with poor outcomes.[6] Despite the absence of arterial hypertension, plasma creatinine is, nevertheless, increased in some patients. Microangiopathic hemolytic anemia and thrombocytopenia are common and contribute to making the diagnosis.[10]

EPIDEMIOLOGY
Prevalence

SSc prevalence is poorly known, with disparities among countries. Based on available series, prevalence is 200 cases per million inhabitants in the United States,[11] 260 cases per million inhabitants in Australia,[11,12] 20 to 50 cases per million inhabitants in Asia,[13] and 100 to 200 cases per million inhabitants in Europe.[14,15]

Because the series came from referral centers in which the most severe cases are concentrated, the published data probably overestimate SRC frequency. Most patients also have limited forms of SSc, without visceral involvement, which are followed in outpatient clinics and are not included in hospital series. As stated above, SRC was more frequent in the 1970s, reaching 19.5% in one series,[16] when ACEIs were not available. At present, SRC occurrence is estimated at 4% to 6% of SSc patients,[17,18] predominantly those with dcSSc. According to classification criteria, SRC was more frequent in dcSSc (12%) than limited cutaneous (lc) SSc (2%) (P<.001) in a single center.[10]

Predictive Factors

Some factors predicting SRC have been described.[19] SRC usually occurs less than 4 years after SSc onset and is more frequently associated dcSSc: the SSc-to-SRC interval was less than 1 year for 66% of the patients according to Penn and colleagues[10] and 3.2 years in the present study.[8]

Anemia, recent cardiac involvement (eg, pericardial effusion, myocarditis with or without congestive heart failure, rhythm and conduction disturbances), and the presence of anti-RNA polymerase III antibodies are signs that SRC could occur, and the use of corticosteroids (CSs; prednisone dose >15–20 mg/d) is a risk factor. In the authors' study,[8] more SRC patients had taken CSs before or concomitantly with SRC onset than SSc patients without past history of SRC used as controls: 64 (70.3%) versus 156 (36.5%) (P<.001), respectively; treated SRC patients had received significantly more CSs than controls (mean ± SD: 29.3 ± 28.4 vs 3.6 ± 9.9 mg, respectively; P<.001). In their case-control study, Steen and Medsger[20] also found that exposure to high-dose CSs (≥15 mg/d of prednisone or its equivalent) during the 6 months preceding SRC onset or the first medical consultation was more frequent among SRC patients than controls (36% vs 12%). Thus, CSs might play a role in triggering SRC. In line with those data, high-dose CSs should be avoided in patients at risk of SRC. In addition, SRC onset after cyclosporin has been reported.

Pre-existing hypertension, proteinuria, elevated serum creatinine, antitopoisomerase-1 (Scl-70), or anticentromere antibodies and histologic abnormalities in renal blood vessels before SRC onset have not been shown to be associated with an increased SRC frequency.

SRC may also develop in kidney-transplant recipients in the context of SSc end-stage renal disease.[21] SRC predictors have been identified and include early native renal function loss following SSc onset, and the clinical markers usually associated with severe disease, like progression of diffuse skin thickening, anemia, and cardiac manifestations.

PATHOPHYSIOLOGY

SRC pathophysiology is incompletely understood,[22] and pathogenic mechanisms are multiple, complex, and interconnected.

Blood-Flow Reduction

The primary cause remains unknown but starts in the renal vascular intima, causing narrowing of vessel lumens and reduced blood flow.[23] Local vasoconstriction, resembling "Raynaud phenomenon," participates in the decreased renal perfusion.[24] Indeed, a higher SRC frequency observed in winter in a large series could support that hypothesis.[4] Cortical blood flow was significantly decreased in patients with SRC or progressive renal failure, whereas it was normal in SSc patients without renal involvement.[25] However, Doppler ultrasonography and renal scintigraphy, which can measure blood flow, failed to identify patients at risk for developing SRC.[25,26] The presence of onion bulbs around the vessels in kidney biopsies could reflect the underlying intimal involvement.

The Renin-Angiotensin-Aldosterone System Involvement

Among other mechanisms, activation of the renin-angiotensin-aldosterone system plays a major role.[27] The renovascular process is responsible for arterial hypertension. Plasma renin is extremely high, and juxtaglomerular apparatus hyperplasia has been found at autopsy.[28] As for every cause of renovascular arterial hypertension, hormone levels are elevated but not correlated with its severity or SRC occurrence.[19,29]

Endothelin

Among SSc symptoms, SRC can be considered part of the renal vasculopathy, along with other clinical manifestations: pulmonary arterial hypertension, Raynaud phenomenon, digital ulcers. Endothelin-1 (ET-1) has been shown to be involved SSc vascular manifestations.[30–32]

Higher circulating ET-1 levels were documented in SSc patients with SRC and in those with pulmonary arterial hypertension.[33,34] Several authors detected the expression of ET-1[35] and ET-1 receptors A and B in kidney biopsies of patients with SRC.[34,35]

Because vascular changes and hyperreninemia may be present in asymptomatic SSc patients, additional factors are probably involved in triggering SRC. Thus, several other factors responsible for reduced renal blood flow (eg, sepsis, dehydration, cardiac arrhythmia, and congestive heart failure)[19] might trigger SRC onset. In addition, the role of pregnancy per se is debated.[36,37]

Drugs

Many substances (eg, cocaine[38]) and drugs, including cyclosporin[39] and CSs,[20,40–42] have been implicated in precipitating SRC. In a case-controlled study, during the 6 months before SRC onset or to the first consultation, high-dose CSs (prednisone: $\geq$15 mg/d) were taken significantly more frequently by SRC patients (36%) than controls (12%) (odds ratio [OR]: 4.37).[20] The authors recently reported on a cohort of 91 SSc patients who developed SRC: 70% of them had been exposed to CSs before

SRC and 56 were taking CSs at the time of SRC onset.[8] In another personal study, the respective ORs for developing SRC associated with CS exposure during the preceding 3- or 1-month periods were 24.1 and 17.4, respectively.[42] Helfrich and colleagues[40] also observed an association between high-dose CSs (>30 mg/d) and normotensive SRC. CS responsibility in SRC occurrence now seems to be established, even though CSs were mainly prescribed for severe dcSSc, a condition favoring SRC.

The mechanism by which CSs might trigger SRC has not yet been clearly identified. ET-1 might be involved, because elevated circulating ET-1 levels were documented in SSc patients with SRC and those with pulmonary arterial hypertension.[33,34]

CLINICAL FEATURES

The main clinical characteristics of patients experiencing SRC reported in published cohorts are listed in **Table 1**.[8,10,41,43] Most patients, around 90%, are hypertensive, and symptoms of malignant hypertension are usually observed. Clinical signs are hypertensive encephalopathy with headache, congestive heart failure, and arrhythmia.

Table 1
Main clinical and biological manifestations of scleroderma renal crisis

Manifestation	Steen,[9] 2003	Walker et al,[43] 2003	DeMarco et al,[41] 2002	Penn et al,[10] 2007	Guillevin et al,[8] 2012
Number of patients	145	16	18	110	91
Mean age, y	50	54	45	51	50
Sex, % men	25	31	17	21	24
Symptoms <4 y, %	76	69	100	66 (<1 y)	79 (<3 y)
dcSSc, %	83	100	100	78	86
AntiScl-70 antibodies, %	20	6	NR	17	31
Anticentromere antibodies, %	1	0	NR	1.8	0
Hypertension, %	90	94	NR	NR	86
Blood pressure, mm Hg	184/108	203/113	130/76	193/114	189/111
Pericarditis, %	53	NR	NR	NR	38
Cardiac insufficiency, %	25	56	39	31	46
Arrhythmia, %	NR	NR	NR	NR	NR
Seizures, %	8	12	NR	NR	NR
Hypertensive encephalopathy, %	NR	NR	NR	NR	58
Thrombotic microangiopathy, %	30	81	NR	59	56
Platelet count <150,000/mm^3, %	39	NR	NR	50	NR
Hematuria, %	38	NR	NR	NR	42[a]
Proteinuria, %	63 (>0.25 g/d)	NR	NR	NR	53 (>0.5 g/d)

Abbreviation: NR, not reported.
[a] Hematuria documented with dipstick or urinalysis.

Hypertensive encephalopathy is characterized by acute or subacute onset of lethargy, fatigue, confusion, headaches, perturbed vision (blurring and exceptionally blindness), and seizures. It is extremely severe but has the advantage of contributing to the diagnosis of SRC. Brain hemorrhage is even rarer. Seizures can be focal or generalized. Congestive heart failure is a common consequence of arterial hypertension. Some patients may have substantial pericardial effusion. Pulmonary hemorrhage has been described and can be life-threatening in some patients.[44,45]

Normotensive Scleroderma Renal Crisis

SRC occurs in 11% to 14% of the patients without hypertension,[8,40] even though some patients develop arterial hypertension later.[10] Patients developing normotensive SRC are often exposed to CSs; two-thirds of them have thrombotic microangiopathy, and their prognoses are worse than when hypertension is present.[40,42]

Distinguishing between SRC with microangiopathy and thrombotic thrombocytopenic microangiopathy usually associated with anti-ADAMTS-13 antibodies is important because their treatments differ. SSc is the direct cause of thrombopathic microangiopathy[46] and is not linked to these autoantibodies. In this setting, assessment of von Willebrand factor protease-cleaving activity might help differentiate these 2 entities.[47] In SSc/SRC, the ADAMTS-13 level is lower than in controls.[48]

Scleroderma Renal Crisis Sine Scleroderma

SRC can occur in patients without skin sclerosis, usually during the year following disease onset.[49,50] Clinical features are recent onset of Raynaud phenomenon, fatigue, weight loss, polyarthritis, swollen hands, carpal tunnel syndrome, and tendon-friction rubs. After a few months of evolution, the skin on the hands and fingers thickens, and thickening spreads proximally to arms, legs, and trunk.

Pregnancy and Scleroderma Renal Crisis

Whether the risk of SRC is increased during pregnancy remains a matter of debate.[37] Indeed, it is sometimes difficult to distinguish pre-eclampsia from SRC in pregnant SSc patients. Importantly, renal function is usually normal in pre-eclampsia. Elevated liver enzymes may orient the diagnosis toward eclampsia or HELLP (hemolysis, elevated liver enzymes, low platelets) syndrome.

For patients with a history of SRC, there is a tendency to consider pregnancy contraindicated. However, it is difficult to offer a global recommendation, and a patient-tailored strategy is probably required. Thus, for a woman with normal renal function and controlled hypertension, pregnancy may probably be attempted. However, whether ACEIs, which are contraindicated during the second and third trimesters of pregnancy, should be interrupted remains a matter of debate.

Differential Diagnosis

SRC is not the sole cause of renal insufficiency or renal involvement. Based on the series by Steen and colleagues[16] of 675 SSc patients, 19.5% developed SRC, 48% had no renal involvement, and 29% experienced other-cause kidney involvements. Atherosclerosis is one of the causes of renal involvement, which could become more frequent in the future as a consequence of patient aging. No specific manifestations of SSc-associated atherosclerosis have been reported.

Not coincidentally, antineutrophil cytoplasmic antibody (ANCA) -associated vasculitides (AAVs) have also been observed during the course of SSc. Few studies have investigated the presence and role of ANCA in SSc. The frequency of ANCA positivity in SSc patients with renal manifestations, assessed by immunofluorescence (IF) or enzyme-linked immunosorbent assay (ELISA), ranged from 0% to 11.7%.[51–58] Anti-myeloperoxidase (MPO) antibodies are present more often in SSc patients with renal vasculitis than those directed against proteinase-3. Ruffatti and colleagues[59] conducted a prevalence study using IF and ELISA (antiproteinase 3 [PR3] and anti-MPO) screening tests and found p-ANCA in only 5 of 115 SSc patients, with anti-PR3 antibodies in 2 patients, anti-MPO antibodies in 1 patient, and both antibodies in 2 patients. Quéméneur and colleagues[57] reviewed 9 personal and 37 literature cases; lcSSc was the main subtype, with an immunologic profile marked by a high frequency of antiScl-70 antibodies. Based on their literature review, Rho and colleagues[60] had previously suggested that anti-Scl-70 antibodies could play a role in SSc patients developing AAVs and be a significant predictor of such events. However, SSc was not more severe when associated with AAVs. AAVs were diagnosed a mean 8.1 years after SSc. Twenty-eight percent of patients received D-penicillamine for a median of 5.5 (range: 0–24) years. Seven of the 46 patients were taking D-penicillamine at the time of AAV diagnosis. D-Penicillamine, like other mechanisms, may therefore play a role in AAVs occurring in SSc, as in other diseases.[61] The final diagnoses were microscopic polyangiitis (27/46), renal limited vasculitis (18/46), and others (1/46). Most of the previously reported AAV cases associated with SSc were described as normotensive renal failure. In 1989, Helfrich and colleagues[40] described 15 SSc patients with normotensive renal failure who frequently showed signs of hemolytic anemia and thrombocytopenia; notably, 6 patients with alveolar hemorrhages were thrombocytopenic.

Among other differential diagnoses, renal arterial stenosis at onset can closely resemble SRC. Hypovolemia caused by dehydration in patients with gut involvement, taking diuretics or nonsteroidal anti-inflammatory drugs (NSAIDs), in cardiac failure, or with arrhythmia, can also mimic SRC.

Nephrotic range proteinuria can also be due to NSAID toxicity. Finally, in a prospective observational study, Steen and colleagues[16] observed that only 5% of 675 patients with dcSSc had unexplained renal abnormalities over a mean follow-up of 12.5 years.

Laboratory Findings

Serum creatinine can be markedly increased at SRC onset. Even after controlling blood pressure, serum creatinine can continue to increase for several days. Urinalysis frequently shows moderate proteinuria (0.5–2.5 g/L). Microscopic hematuria, often detected by dipstick, could also correspond to hemoglobinuria in most patients.

Thrombotic microangiopathy, defined as hemolytic anemia and thrombocytopenia, occurs in 43% of SRC patients. Thrombocytopenia is usually moderate, greater than 50,000 platelets/mm^3 for most patients, and frequently returns to within the normal range once blood pressure is controlled.

Antinuclear antibodies are common. Anti-Scl-70 antibodies, detected in 36% of a large Italian patient series,[62] were found more frequently in dcSSc (58.6% in that series) and were not predictive of SRC. Anti-RNA polymerase-III antibodies are rarely present in the French SSc population.[63] They have been detected almost exclusively in early dcSSc, notably with rapidly diffuse skin progression,[64] and 33% of anti-RNA polymerase-III-positive patients will develop SRC.[65] Lower anti-Scl-70 and anticentromere antibody frequencies contrasted with higher anti-RNA polymerase-III frequency in SRC patients. In the authors' series of 91 patients,[8] anti-RNA polymerase-III antibodies were sought in 18 and detected in 27% (29.7% in another series from their group).[66] In the Teixeira study,[42] anticentromere antibodies were found in none of the SRC patients and anti-Scl-70 in were found in 32% of SRC patients.

Anticentromere antibody positivity does not totally preclude SRC, but they are found in only 1% to 3% of SRC patients,[8,67] making its occurrence improbable.

Thus, when anti-RNA polymerase-III antibodies are present, the potential for SRC should be kept in mind.

Renal Pathology

A persisting major question concerns the necessity and advantages of obtaining a renal biopsy. The authors think that it could be recommended but is certainly not essential. For patients in poor general condition whose clinical and biological profiles are typical, biopsy is not needed or can be delayed until the patient's health status improves. However, renal biopsy offers some advantages: exclusion of differential diagnoses, diagnosis confirmation, and evaluation of prognosis based on kidney histology.[10,68] For atypical forms, renal biopsy becomes mandatory to confirm SRC diagnosis. For some patients, renal biopsy should be obtained only after blood pressure is controlled, giving clinicians the time to decide whether to biopsy. When thrombocytopenia is severe, renal biopsy should not be performed or can be done through jugular vein catheterization.

The histologic lesions are vascular, glomerular, tubular, and interstitial.

Vessels

The ischemic process can be responsible for renal infarcts and subcapsular hemorrhages.[69] Lesions are similar to those observed in malignant hypertension (ie, predominantly affecting intralobular arteries and arterioles). Arcuate arteries can also be involved. Larger arteries are normal or exhibit nonspecific anomalies. Vessel-wall modifications concern the endothelium, with mucoid intimal thickening and myointimal cellular proliferation without inflammatory cells. The mucinous intimal change mostly consists of glycoprotein and mucopolysaccharides. Fibrinoid deposits and, sometimes, fibrinoid necrosis may be seen in the arterial wall, mainly in the intima, without vasculitis, resulting in vessel-lumen narrowing and occlusion.[70] In some patients, the presence of arteriolar fibrinoid necrosis or thrombosis indicates thrombotic microangiopathy. Notably, unlike lesions encountered in malignant hypertension without SSc, the media of interlobular arteries are often thinned and surrounded by periadventitial and adventitial fibroses.

Glomeruli

Glomerular changes are common, usually focal, but glomeruli can be normal or ischemic with flocculus retraction. The juxtaglomerular apparatus is clearly seen and may be hyperplastic, reflecting its hyperactivity, causing hyperreninemia that can occur during SRC.[28] Immunoglobulin (Ig) and complement deposits are not specific; IgM, IgG, IgA, C3, or C1q may be detected in small arteries, arterioles, glomeruli, or mesangium. However, it is important to note that many of these histologic changes can also be observed in SSc patients who do not develop SRC or in patients with malignant hypertension without SSc.

Tubular and interstitial lesions

Ischemia can affect the tubular epithelium, causing acute multifocal tubular necrosis. Interstitial lesions are nonspecific.

Outcomes and Prognoses

SRC outcomes reported for the largest published series are detailed in **Table 2**. Before the 1980s and the advent of ACEIs, SRC almost always resulted in renal failure and death, usually within months. The use of ACEIs has dramatically improved SRC

Table 2
Outcomes of scleroderma renal crisis

Parameter	Steen & Medsger,[6] 2000	Walker et al,[43] 2003	DeMarco et al,[41] 2002	Penn et al,[10] 2007	Teixeira et al,[42] 2008	Guillevin et al,[8] 2012
Number of patients	145[a]	16	18	110	50	91
Dialyzed patients, %	62	31	NR	64	56	54
Temporarily, %	23	6	NR	23	16	22
Permanently, %	19	25	NR	42	22	78[b]
Died on dialysis, %	NR	NR	NR	18	18	44
Dead at 5 y, %	19[c]	31	50	41	31	60

Abbreviation: NR, not reported.
[a] All patients were treated with ACEIs.
[b] Permanently dialyzed or died.
[c] Early deaths.

prognosis.[6] Steen and Medsger[6] reported good outcomes for 60% of the patients who participated in the largest prospective observational cohort study to date,[71] with 15% 1-year mortality for those not given ACEIs.[71] Conversely, among 76% of those patients who had received ACEIs and were alive at 1 year, only 10% survived at 5 years.[71] Penn and colleagues[10] reported 1-, 2-, 3-, 5-, and 10-year survival rates of 82%, 74%, 71%, 59%, and 47%, respectively. In the authors' study,[8] respective 1-, 2-, 5-, and 10-year survival rates for SRC patients were 70.9%, 66.6%, 60%, and 41.9%.

Steen and colleagues[6,71] identified risk factors associated with poor outcomes: male sex, older age, congestive heart failure, serum creatinine greater than 3 mg/dL at treatment onset, and greater than 3 days required to control blood pressure. The survival rate was lower for dialyzed patients versus no dialysis, and patients whose renal function improved and came off dialysis had better outcomes than those who were dialyzed and those never dialyzed (**Fig. 1**).[10] Dialysis is usually required early, at SRC onset, and much less frequently for patients developing SRC later on. However, the severity of the glomerular ischemic process can be responsible for progressive renal function deterioration, affecting 4%, according to Steen and Medsger.[6]

Finally, according to the recent prospective international study,[72] 36% of SRC patients had died by 1 year, which is higher than had been found in retrospective analyses.[8,10] Thus, retrospective studies probably missed incident SRC cases, and future prospective SSc investigations will provide better understanding of the natural history of SRC onset and its real outcomes.

Overall, however, it is important to note that the long-term outcomes of patients who survived the first year of SRC not on dialysis are somewhat better.

Treatment

SRC treatment combines drug treatment and management of severely ill patients in intensive care units or renal departments. Over the long term, treatments include not only managing end-stage renal failure, dialysis, and transplantation, but also the general care of severe dcSSc. SRC patients are usually in poor general condition and often have SRC sequelae that can be difficult to handle.

Drugs

ACEIs are the main SRC treatment. Before the widespread use of this family of drugs, outcomes were poor and mortality was high.[71] Angiotensin II (ATII) -receptor inhibitors

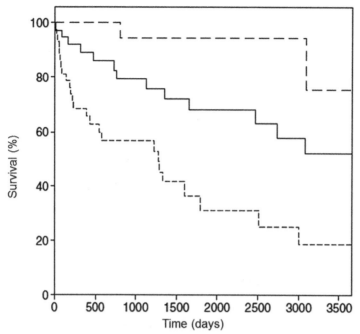

Fig. 1. Survival after SRC by renal outcome: no dialysis (—), dialysis and recovery of renal function (– – –), or dialysis without recovered renal function (- - -). (*From* Penn H, Howie AJ, Kingdon EJ, et al. Scleroderma renal crisis: patient characteristics and long-term outcomes. QJM 2007;100(8):490; with permission.)

have also been proposed. For unexplained reasons, responses to ACEIs or ATII-receptor inhibitor are not good in all patients,[43,73] perhaps reflecting heterogeneity of genetic polymorphisms in SSc patients,[74] but that has not been evaluated in patients with and without SRC.

ACEIs must be prescribed to all SSc-SRC patients, even those with impaired renal function. A short-acting ACEI is recommended (eg, captopril at 6.5 to 12.5 mg every 8 hours). The dose can be progressively increased, until blood pressure normalizes and renal function improves. Treatment goals are blood pressure control and improved renal function. Up to half of the patients require dialysis. Once an ACEI has been started and is effective, renal function usually stabilizes. Other antihypertensive drugs can be added to an ACEI if SRC does not respond to treatment. Vasodilators, like calcium-channel blockers, are the drugs of choice. β-Blockers should not be prescribed, except to patients with cardiac insufficiency, where they can improve cardiac function. Labetalol can be prescribed.

In SRC patients with normal blood pressure, an ACEI can also be prescribed but careful blood pressure, volemia status, and renal function monitoring is necessary.

Adjunct therapy with continuous low doses of prostacyclin has been recommended,[18] without strong evidence that it improved short- and long-term SRC prognoses. Plasma exchange, which has been proposed for thrombotic microangiopathy, has not demonstrated efficacy and should not be prescribed, with the exception of the rare SRC patients who might develop thrombotic microangiopathy associated with anti-ADAMTS-13 antibodies (Mouthon and colleagues, unpublished data).

Based on ET-1 detection in the kidney biopsies of SRC patients, ET-receptor blockers were combined with an ACEI and recently found to have acceptable tolerance in a small, open study.[75] Serum ET-1 was elevated in SRC patients, compared with healthy controls (P<.0005), and ET-1 and ET-1 receptors A and B were strongly expressed in the biopsied SRC patients.[75] Additional prospective studies are needed to document the efficacy of anti-ET-1 receptor antagonists combined with an ACEI during the acute phase of SRC in a larger patient cohort, with close follow-up, particularly for intermediate- and long-term effects. In this setting, the authors are conducting a prospective multicenter open study, ReinBO, on 16 SRC patients taking an ACEI for 6 months in whom they are analyzing the effect of concomitant ET-1 receptor antagonist bosentan on SRC outcome.

CSs are contraindicated and cytotoxic drugs have not been proven effective as SRC treatment.

Dialysis and transplantation

Long-term dialysis increases the risk of death. Independently of the underlying disease, dialysis increases the risk of infection (in patients undergoing peritoneal dialysis) and, over the long term, enhances the risk of atherosclerosis and vascular diseases. In patients on chronic dialysis, kidney transplantation has to be considered. The final decision to transplant should not be made before 2 years after SRC onset. For a series of 260 SSc patients who underwent renal transplantation in the United States, their 5-year graft-survival rate was 56.7%.[21] In that study, the risk of SRC recurrence was higher for patients with early renal insufficiency following SRC onset. Recurrent SRC in the allograft may be predicted by the same previously described risk factors.[21] For those with recurrent SRC, the time of onset following transplantation is not known. Recurrence usually happens within the first few months to the first 1 to 2 years after transplantation.[21]

Prevention

Montanelli and colleagues[76] recently reported their retrospective analysis of 410 SSc patients with disease duration less than 5 years whose risk of developing SRC was sharply reduced for those prescribed calcium-channel blockers. The use of prophylactic ACEIs remains a matter of debate, because some SSc patients developed SRC while taking these agents.[18,42,77] Usually, patients given an ACEI for SRC continue this treatment with no recommendation to stop it. ACEIs have been proposed to treat other vascular manifestations in SSc patients. They provided no benefit against Raynaud phenomenon or digital ulcers in the QUINS trial (quinapril)[78] that was conducted on patients with lcSSc or Raynaud phenomenon associated with antinuclear antibodies. The use of an ACEI/ATII-receptor antagonist before SRC was associated with somewhat poorer outcomes in retrospective studies on dialyzed patients.[10,42] Analysis of pooled data from those 2 studies yielded an OR of 2.4 (P = .059; χ^2 = 3.64).[10] Thus, whether a low-dose prophylactic ACEI protects against SRC or leads to increased risk of more severe SRC remains a matter of controversy. In a recent, prospective, observational, Web-based cohort study on 88 patients with incident SRC, including 13 lost to follow-up, 18 (24%) had received an ACEI immediately before SRC onset. According to unadjusted analyses, ACEI exposure before SRC onset was associated with an increased risk of death (hazard ratio 2.42, 95% CI 1.02–5.75; P<.05 in the primary analysis and 2.17, 95% CI 0.88–5.33; P = .09 after post-hoc adjustment for pre-existing hypertension). However, as stated by the investigators, the wide confidence intervals, indicating considerable uncertainty around the precise magnitude of the risk and the possibility of residual confounding, remained important limitations.[72] Those results need further confirmation, ideally from a randomized controlled trial on a large sample of patients.

SUMMARY

SRC is a rare complication of SSc that remains severe. Prompt recognition and initiation of therapy with an ACEI offer the best chance to achieve a good outcome. Nevertheless, 5-year mortality remains unacceptably high, and other therapeutic strategies are needed to improve the prognosis.

REFERENCES

1. Gabrielli A, Avvedimento EV, Krieg T. Scleroderma. N Engl J Med 2009;360(19): 1989–2003.
2. Steen VD. The many faces of scleroderma. Rheum Dis Clin North Am 2008;34(1): 1–15, v.
3. Moore HC, Sheehan HL. The kidney of scleroderma. Lancet 1952;1(6698):68–70.
4. Traub YM, Shapiro AP, Rodnan GP, et al. Hypertension and renal failure (scleroderma renal crisis) in progressive systemic sclerosis. Review of a 25-year experience with 68 cases. Medicine (Baltimore) 1983;62(6):335–52.
5. Hunzelmann N, Genth E, Krieg T, et al. The registry of the German Network for Systemic Scleroderma: frequency of disease subsets and patterns of organ involvement. Rheumatology (Oxford) 2008;47(8):1185–92.
6. Steen VD, Medsger TA Jr. Long-term outcomes of scleroderma renal crisis. Ann Intern Med 2000;133(8):600–3.
7. Steen VD, Medsger TA Jr. Severe organ involvement in systemic sclerosis with diffuse scleroderma. Arthritis Rheum 2000;43(11):2437–44.
8. Guillevin L, Berezne A, Seror R, et al. Scleroderma renal crisis: a retrospective multicentre study on 91 patients and 427 controls. Rheumatology (Oxford) 2012;51(3):460–7.
9. Steen VD. Scleroderma renal crisis. Rheum Dis Clin North Am 2003;29(2):315–33.
10. Penn H, Howie AJ, Kingdon EJ, et al. Scleroderma renal crisis: patient characteristics and long-term outcomes. QJM 2007;100(8):485–94.
11. Mayes MD, Lacey JV Jr, Beebe-Dimmer J, et al. Prevalence, incidence, survival, and disease characteristics of systemic sclerosis in a large US population. Arthritis Rheum 2003;48(8):2246–55.
12. Roberts-Thomson PJ, Walker JG. Scleroderma: it has been a long hard journey. Intern Med J 2006;36(8):519–23.
13. Tamaki T, Mori S, Takehara K. Epidemiological study of patients with systemic sclerosis in Tokyo. Arch Dermatol Res 1991;283(6):366–71.
14. Le Guern V, Mahr A, Mouthon L, et al. Prevalence of systemic sclerosis in a French multi-ethnic county. Rheumatology (Oxford) 2004;43(9):1129–37.
15. Magnant J, Diot E. Sclerodermie systemique: epidemiologie et facteurs environnementaux. Presse Med 2006;35(12 Pt 2):1894–901.
16. Steen VD, Syzd A, Johnson JP, et al. Kidney disease other than renal crisis in patients with diffuse scleroderma. J Rheumatol 2005;32(4):649–55.
17. Walker UA, Tyndall A, Czirjak L, et al. Clinical risk assessment of organ manifestations in systemic sclerosis: a report from the EULAR Scleroderma Trials And Research group database. Ann Rheum Dis 2007;66(6):754–63.
18. Denton CP, Black CM. Scleroderma–clinical and pathological advances. Best Pract Res Clin Rheumatol 2004;18(3):271–90.
19. Steen VD, Medsger TA Jr, Osial TA Jr, et al. Factors predicting development of renal involvement in progressive systemic sclerosis. Am J Med 1984;76(5): 779–86.

20. Steen VD, Medsger TA. Case-control study of corticosteroids and other drugs that either precipitate or protect from the development of scleroderma renal crisis. Arthritis Rheum 1998;41(9):1613–9.

21. Pham PT, Pham PC, Danovitch GM, et al. Predictors and risk factors for recurrent scleroderma renal crisis in the kidney allograft: case report and review of the literature. Am J Transplant 2005;5(10):2565–9.

22. Denton CP, Lapadula G, Mouthon L, et al. Renal complications and scleroderma renal crisis. Rheumatology (Oxford) 2009;48(Suppl 3):iii32–5.

23. Charles C, Clements P, Furst DE. Systemic sclerosis: hypothesis-driven treatment strategies. Lancet 2006;367(9523):1683–91.

24. Cannon PJ, Hassar M, Case DB, et al. The relationship of hypertension and renal failure in scleroderma (progressive systemic sclerosis) to structural and functional abnormalities of the renal cortical circulation. Medicine (Baltimore) 1974; 53(1):1–46.

25. Rivolta R, Mascagni B, Berruti V, et al. Renal vascular damage in systemic sclerosis patients without clinical evidence of nephropathy. Arthritis Rheum 1996; 39(6):1030–4.

26. Woolfson RG, Cairns HS, Williams DJ, et al. Renal scintigraphy in acute scleroderma: report of three cases. J Nucl Med 1993;34(7):1163–5.

27. Gavras H, Gavras I, Cannon PJ, et al. Is elevated plasma renin activity of prognostic importance in progressive systemic sclerosis? Arch Intern Med 1977; 137(11):1554–8.

28. Stone RA, Tisher CC, Hawkins HK, et al. Juxtaglomerular hyperplasia and hyperreninemia in progressive systemic sclerosis complicated acute renal failure. Am J Med 1974;56(1):119–23.

29. Clements PJ, Lachenbruch PA, Furst DE, et al. Abnormalities of renal physiology in systemic sclerosis. A prospective study with 10-year followup. Arthritis Rheum 1994;37(1):67–74.

30. Guillevin L. Translating ideas into progress in systemic sclerosis. Rheumatology (Oxford) 2009;48(Suppl 3):iii58–60.

31. Mayes MD. Endothelin and endothelin receptor antagonists in systemic rheumatic disease. Arthritis Rheum 2003;48(5):1190–9.

32. Koch AE, Distler O. Vasculopathy and disordered angiogenesis in selected rheumatic diseases: rheumatoid arthritis and systemic sclerosis. Arthritis Res Ther 2007;9(Suppl 2):S3.

33. Vancheeswaran R, Magoulas T, Efrat G, et al. Circulating endothelin-1 levels in systemic sclerosis subsets–a marker of fibrosis or vascular dysfunction? J Rheumatol 1994;21(10):1838–44.

34. Kobayashi H, Nishimaki T, Kaise S, et al. Immunohistological study endothelin-1 and endothelin-A and B receptors in two patients with scleroderma renal crisis. Clin Rheumatol 1999;18(5):425–7.

35. Mouthon L, Mehrenberger M, Teixeira L, et al. Endothelin-1 expression in scleroderma renal crisis. Hum Pathol 2011;42(1):95–102.

36. Steen VD, Conte C, Day N, et al. Pregnancy in women with systemic sclerosis. Arthritis Rheum 1989;32(2):151–7.

37. Steen VD. Pregnancy in women with systemic sclerosis. Obstet Gynecol 1999; 94(1):15–20.

38. Lam M, Ballou SP. Reversible scleroderma renal crisis after cocaine use. N Engl J Med 1992;326(21):1435.

39. Denton CP, Sweny P, Abdulla A, et al. Acute renal failure occurring in scleroderma treated with cyclosporin A: a report of three cases. Br J Rheumatol 1994;33(1):90–2.

40. Helfrich DJ, Banner B, Steen VD, et al. Normotensive renal failure in systemic sclerosis. Arthritis Rheum 1989;32(9):1128–34.

41. DeMarco PJ, Weisman MH, Seibold JR, et al. Predictors and outcomes of scleroderma renal crisis: the high-dose versus low-dose D-penicillamine in early diffuse systemic sclerosis trial. Arthritis Rheum 2002;46(11):2983–9.

42. Teixeira L, Mouthon L, Mahr A, et al. Mortality and risk factors of scleroderma renal crisis: a French retrospective study of 50 patients. Ann Rheum Dis 2008; 67(1):110–6.

43. Walker J, Ahern M, Smith M, et al. Scleroderma renal crisis: poor outcome despite aggressive antihypertensive treatment. Intern Med J 2003;33(5–6):216–20.

44. Herndon TM, Kim TT, Goeckeritz BE, et al. Alveolar hemorrhage and pulmonary hypertension in systemic sclerosis: a continuum of scleroderma renal crisis? J Clin Rheumatol 2001;7(2):115–9.

45. Naniwa T, Banno S, Takahashi N, et al. Normotensive scleroderma renal crisis with diffuse alveolar damage after corticosteroid therapy. Mod Rheumatol 2005; 15(2):134–8.

46. George JN, Nester CM. Syndromes of thrombotic microangiopathy. N Engl J Med 2014;371(7):654–66.

47. Manadan AM, Harris C, Block JA. Thrombotic thrombocytopenic purpura in the setting of systemic sclerosis. Semin Arthritis Rheum 2005;34(4):683–8.

48. Mannucci PM, Vanoli M, Forza I, et al. Von Willebrand factor cleaving protease (ADAMTS-13) in 123 patients with connective tissue diseases (systemic lupus erythematosus and systemic sclerosis). Haematologica 2003;88(8):914–8.

49. Molina JF, Anaya JM, Cabrera GE, et al. Systemic sclerosis sine scleroderma: an unusual presentation in scleroderma renal crisis. J Rheumatol 1995;22(3):557–60.

50. Gonzalez EA, Schmulbach E, Bastani B. Scleroderma renal crisis with minimal skin involvement and no serologic evidence of systemic sclerosis. Am J Kidney Dis 1994;23(2):317–9.

51. Avouac J, Airo P, Dieude P, et al. Associated autoimmune diseases in systemic sclerosis define a subset of patients with milder disease: results from 2 large cohorts of European Caucasian patients. J Rheumatol 2010;37(3):608–14.

52. Carvajal I, Bernis C, Sanz P, et al. Antineutrophil cytoplasmic autoantibodies (ANCA) and systemic sclerosis. Nephrol Dial Transplant 1997;12(3):576–7.

53. Locke IC, Worrall JG, Leaker B, et al. Autoantibodies to myeloperoxidase in systemic sclerosis. J Rheumatol 1997;24(1):86–9.

54. Maes B, Van Mieghem A, Messiaen T, et al. Limited cutaneous systemic sclerosis associated with MPO-ANCA positive renal small vessel vasculitis of the microscopic polyangiitis type. Am J Kidney Dis 2000;36(3):E16.

55. Merkel PA, Polisson RP, Chang Y, et al. Prevalence of antineutrophil cytoplasmic antibodies in a large inception cohort of patients with connective tissue disease. Ann Intern Med 1997;126(11):866–73.

56. Mimura I, Hori Y, Matsukawa T, et al. Noncrescentic ANCA-associated renal crisis in systemic sclerosis. Clin Nephrol 2008;70(2):183–5.

57. Quéméneur T, Mouthon L, Cacoub P, et al. Systemic vasculitis during the course of systemic sclerosis: report of 12 cases and review of the literature. Medicine (Baltimore) 2013;92(1):1–9.

58. Derrett-Smith EC, Nihtyanova SI, Harvey J, et al. Revisiting ANCA-associated vasculitis in systemic sclerosis: clinical, serological and immunogenetic factors. Rheumatology (Oxford) 2013;52(10):1824–31.

59. Ruffatti A, Sinico RA, Radice A, et al. Autoantibodies to proteinase 3 and myeloperoxidase in systemic sclerosis. J Rheumatol 2002;29(5):918–23.

60. Rho YH, Choi SJ, Lee YH, et al. Scleroderma associated with ANCA-associated vasculitis. Rheumatol Int 2006;26(5):369–75.
61. Bienaime F, Clerbaux G, Plaisier E, et al. D-Penicillamine-induced ANCA-associated crescentic glomerulonephritis in Wilson disease. Am J Kidney Dis 2007;50(5):821–5.
62. Ferri C, Valentini G, Cozzi F, et al. Systemic sclerosis: demographic, clinical, and serologic features and survival in 1,012 Italian patients. Medicine (Baltimore) 2002;81(2):139–53.
63. Faucher B, Stein P, Granel B, et al. Low prevalence of anti-RNA polymerase III antibodies in a French scleroderma population: anti-RNA polymerase III sclero-derma. Eur J Intern Med 2010;21(2):114–7.
64. Cavazzana I, Angela C, Paolo A, et al. Anti-RNA polymerase III antibodies: a marker of systemic sclerosis with rapid onset and skin thickening progression. Autoimmun Rev 2009;8(7):580–4.
65. Okano Y, Steen VD, Medsger TA Jr. Autoantibody reactive with RNA polymerase III in systemic sclerosis. Ann Intern Med 1993;119(10):1005–13.
66. Emilie S, Goulvestre C, Berezne A, et al. Anti-RNA polymerase III antibodies are associated with scleroderma renal crisis in a French cohort. Scand J Rheumatol 2011;40(5):404–6.
67. Steen V. Renal involvement in systemic sclerosis. In: Clements PJ, Furst D, editors. Systemic sclerosis. 2nd edition. Lippincott; 2004. p. 279–92.
68. Penn H, Denton CP. Diagnosis, management and prevention of scleroderma renal disease. Curr Opin Rheumatol 2008;20(6):692–6.
69. Fisher ER, Rodnan GP. Pathologic observations concerning the kidney in progressive systemic sclerosis. AMA Arch Pathol 1958;65(1):29–39.
70. Trostle DC, Bedetti CD, Steen VD, et al. Renal vascular histology and morphometry in systemic sclerosis. A case-control autopsy study. Arthritis Rheum 1988; 31(3):393–400.
71. Steen VD, Costantino JP, Shapiro AP, et al. Outcome of renal crisis in systemic sclerosis: relation to availability of angiotensin converting enzyme (ACE) inhibitors. Ann Intern Med 1990;113(5):352–7.
72. Hudson M, Baron M, Tatibouet S, et al. Exposure to ACE inhibitors prior to the onset of scleroderma renal crisis-results from the International Scleroderma Renal Crisis Survey. Semin Arthritis Rheum 2014;43(5):666–72.
73. Caskey FJ, Thacker EJ, Johnston PA, et al. Failure of losartan to control blood pressure in scleroderma renal crisis. Lancet 1997;349(9052):620.
74. Fatini C, Gensini F, Sticchi E, et al. High prevalence of polymorphisms of angiotensin-converting enzyme (I/D) and endothelial nitric oxide synthase (Glu298Asp) in patients with systemic sclerosis. Am J Med 2002;112(7):540–4.
75. Penn H, Quillinan N, Khan K, et al. Targeting the endothelin axis in scleroderma renal crisis: rationale and feasibility. QJM 2013;106(9):839–48.
76. Montanelli G, Beretta L, Santaniello A, et al. Effect of dihydropyridine calcium channel blockers and glucocorticoids on the prevention and development of scleroderma renal crisis in an Italian case series. Clin Exp Rheumatol 2013; 31(2 Suppl 76):135–9.
77. Steen VD, Medsger TA. Changes in causes of death in systemic sclerosis, 1972–2002. Ann Rheum Dis 2007;66(7):940–4.
78. Maddison P. Prevention of vascular damage in scleroderma with angiotensin-converting enzyme (ACE) inhibition. Rheumatology (Oxford) 2002;41(9):965–71.

Monitoring and Diagnostic Approaches for Pulmonary Arterial Hypertension in Patients with Systemic Sclerosis

CrossMark

Antonia Valenzuela, MD, MS[a], Saranya Nandagopal, BA[b],
Virginia D. Steen, MD[c], Lorinda Chung, MD, MS[d],*

KEYWORDS

- Systemic sclerosis • Pulmonary arterial hypertension • Monitoring • Diagnosis

KEY POINTS

- Pulmonary arterial hypertension (PAH) is one of the leading causes of death in patients with systemic sclerosis (SSc).
- Known risk factors for the development of SSc-PAH are older age, longer disease duration, a low carbon monoxide diffusion in the lung, a low diffusing capacity of carbon monoxide, and high forced vital capacity/diffusing capacity of carbon monoxide.
- Given the high prevalence and poor survival of SSc-PAH, and that aggressive management of mild disease may be associated with better outcomes, screening is critical.
- Right heart catheterization (RHC) is the gold standard for the definitive diagnosis of PAH, and should be performed in those patients in whom this diagnosis is suspected.
- Once a diagnosis of PAH is confirmed by RHC, treatment with PAH-specific therapies should be initiated as soon as possible.

Disclosures: L. Chung has received research support funding from Gilead, United Therapeutics, Pfizer, and Actelion, has served on the Advisory Board for Gilead (<$10,000 per year), and receives funding from the Scleroderma Research Foundation and the Scleroderma Foundation. V.D. Steen has received research support from Gilead, United Therapeutics, and Actelion, has served on Advisory Boards for Gilead and Bayer, and is on the speakers bureau for Actelion and Gilead (<$10,000 per year).

[a] Department of Immunology and Rheumatology, Stanford University School of Medicine, 1000 Welch Road, Suite 203, MC 5755, Palo Alto, CA 94304, USA; [b] Department of Dermatology, Stanford University School of Medicine, 450 Broadway Street, Pavilion C, 2nd Floor, Redwood City, CA 94063, USA; [c] Division of Rheumatology, Allergy, and Immunology, Georgetown University School of Medicine, Pasquerilla Health Center, 6th Floor 3800 Reservoir Road NW, Washington, DC 20007, USA; [d] Department of Immunology and Rheumatology, Stanford University School of Medicine, 1000 Welch Road, Suite 203, MC 5755, Palo Alto, CA 94304, USA
* Corresponding author.
E-mail address: shauwei@stanford.edu

Rheum Dis Clin N Am 41 (2015) 489–506
http://dx.doi.org/10.1016/j.rdc.2015.04.009
0889-857X/15/$ – see front matter Published by Elsevier Inc.

INTRODUCTION

Pulmonary arterial hypertension (PAH) is one of the leading causes of death in patients with systemic sclerosis (SSc). Novel screening approaches, biomarkers, monitoring indices, and PAH-specific treatments have improved prognosis for patients with SSc-PAH, but outcomes are still poor and are worse than for patients with idiopathic PAH (IPAH) or PAH secondary to other connective tissue diseases (CTDs). This article reviews the evidence regarding monitoring and diagnostic approaches for PAH in SSc.

Epidemiology of Pulmonary Hypertension in Systemic Sclerosis

Pulmonary hypertension (PH) is a serious complication associated with SSc.[1–3] PH is defined as a resting mean pulmonary arterial pressure (mPAP) of 25 mm Hg or greater on right heart catheterization (RHC). PAH, a subgroup of PH, is further distinguished by a pulmonary arterial wedge pressure (PAWP) less than or equal to 15 mm Hg, without chronic hypoxemia from interstitial lung disease (ILD).[4] The classification of PH has evolved over time. During the deliberations of the Dana Point conference on classification, a general consensus was reached and 5 groups of PH were defined.[5] In addition to PAH (group 1), they include PH caused by left heart disease (group 2), PH caused by lung diseases and/or hypoxia (group 3), chronic thromboembolic PH (group 4), and PH with unclear multifactorial causes (group 5).[6] PH in SSc is most frequently attributed to group 1 PAH, but group 3 PH related to ILD and group 2 PH related to diastolic dysfunction have been reported to comprise 20% and 16% of SSc-PH cases, respectively.[5,7] Pulmonary veno-occlusive disease (PVOD) and pulmonary capillary hemangiomatosis are rare causes of PH, designated as group 1'. Small case series and case reports have suggested that both are more common in SSc and CTDs than in IPAH.[8–10] PVOD is characterized by extensive, diffuse, and occlusive fibrosis of postcapillary venous pulmonary vessels. It presents in similar fashion to patients with other forms of PAH, but has higher risk of pulmonary edema, often precipitated by PAH-specific therapy.[11] No specific clinical or hemodynamic characteristics predict this complication.[12]

The prevalence of PAH in SSc by RHC is between 7% and 12%.[1] With the exclusion of patients with severe pulmonary fibrosis and severe left heart disease, a multicenter cohort of patients with SSc in France found a prevalence of PAH of 7.85%.[13] The incidence has been estimated to be 0.61 cases per 100 patient-years.[14] Typically, PAH presents 10 to 15 years after the onset of Raynaud phenomenon, but may occur earlier, particularly in patients with diffuse cutaneous SSc.[15]

Risk Factors for Pulmonary Arterial Hypertension in Systemic Sclerosis

Box 1 summarizes the risk factors associated with developing PAH in SSc, including demographics; physical examination findings; autoantibodies; and findings on pulmonary function tests (PFTs), transthoracic echocardiography (TTE), and RHC.

The risk for PAH in patients with SSc increases with older age.[16,17] In addition, postmenopausal status has been associated with the development of PAH,[18] which is consistent with the results of one small retrospective study that showed that hormone replacement therapy may be protective.[19] Some studies have found that patients with the limited cutaneous subtype of SSc, and longer disease duration, are at higher risk of developing PAH[17,20]; however PAH can also affect patients with diffuse cutaneous involvement and earlier disease (within the first 5 years of diagnosis).[16,21] Vascular phenomena, such as increased number of telangiectasias[22] and digital ulcers,[20] have also been associated with the development of PAH.

Box 1
Risk factors for PAH in SSc

Demographics:

  Longer disease duration

  Older age

  Postmenopausal status

Physical finding:

  Increased number of telangiectasias

  Digital ulcers

Autoantibodies:

  Positive anticentromere antibody

  Positive anti–U1-ribonucleoprotein antibody

  Nucleolar pattern of antinuclear antibody

  Positive antiphospholipid antibodies

  Negative anti–Scl-70 antibody

  Positive AECAs

  Positive anti-AT1R and anti-ETAR antibodies

PFT findings:

  DLCO less than 50% of predicted

  DLCO/AV ratio less than 70% of predicted

  FVC/DLCO ratio greater than 1.6

Echocardiographic findings:

  Increased RVSP rate of greater than 3 mm Hg/y

RHC findings:

  mPAP 21 to 24 mm Hg

  TPG greater than 11 mm Hg

Abbreviations: AECA, anti–endothelial cell antibodies; AT1R, anti–angiotensin receptor type 1; AV, alveolar volume; DLCO, diffusing capacity of carbon monoxide; ETAR, anti–endothelin receptor type A; FVC, forced vital capacity; PFT, pulmonary function test; RVSP, right ventricular systolic pressure; TPG, transpulmonary gradient.

The presence of anticentromere antibody (ACA),[23,24] anti–U1-ribonucleoprotein (RNP),[23,25] nucleolar pattern of antinuclear antibody (ANA),[23,26] and antiphospholipid antibodies,[27] and the absence of anti–Scl-70 antibody[28,29] are associated with a higher risk of SSc-PAH. In addition, some novel antibodies, like anti–endothelial cell antibodies (AECAs),[30,31] anti–angiotensin receptor type 1 (AT1R), and anti–endothelin receptor type A (ETAR) antibodies, are more frequent in SSc-PAH than in other forms of PAH (IPAH, chronic thromboembolic PH, and PH caused by congenital heart diseases), and may play a role in increasing endothelial vascular reactivity and inducing pulmonary vasculopathy in patients with SSc. AT1R and ETAR antibodies have been associated with a 2 to 4-fold increased risk of development of SSc-PAH, and ETAR has also been associated with increased mortality related to SSc-PAH (HR 2.7, 95% CI 1.2–6.1, $P = .0271$).[32]

PFTs can be helpful in assessing the risk for PAH in patients with SSc. An isolated low diffusing capacity of carbon monoxide (DLCO) less than 50% of predicted is considered a risk factor, as confirmed by one case-control study of 106 patients with SSc matched for age, sex, disease duration, and cutaneous subtype.[28] In a large European SSc cohort, a higher threshold for DLCO/alveolar volume (AV) ratio (<70% of predicted) was associated with the development of PAH.[16] A disproportionate decline in the DLCO relative to the forced vital capacity (FVC) as shown by an FVC%/DLCO% ratio greater than 1.6 has also been described as a predictor of the presence of PAH.[33–35]

Although echocardiography may overestimate or underestimate the pulmonary artery pressure, one recent study showed that an increase in the annual rate of change of right ventricular systolic pressure (RVSP) on TTE correlates with high probability to develop PAH over a mean follow-up time of 7.7 years.[36] Compared with patients with a stable RVSP, the relative hazard for the development of PAH was 6.15 (95% CI, 3.58–10.56) for subjects whose RVSP increased at rates of greater than 3 mm Hg/y.

Particular hemodynamic features are also associated with progression to PAH in patients with SSc. In a study of 228 patients with SSc screened for PAH with an RHC, patients with borderline mPAP of 21 to 24 mm Hg or a transpulmonary gradient (TPG; the difference between mPAP and mean PAWP) greater than 11 mm Hg at baseline were more likely to develop PAH in subsequent RHC, with an HR of 3.7 (95% CI, 1.7–8.0) and 7.9 (95% CI, 2.7–23.5), respectively.[37] Similarly, in 206 patients from the pulmonary hypertension assessment and recognition of outcomes in scleroderma (PHAROS) multicenter prospective cohort of patients with SSc at risk for PAH, patients with borderline mPAP were more likely to develop resting PAH than patients with normal mPAP (55% vs 32%) at a mean follow-up of 25.7 months.[38]

Clinical Presentation

Patients with SSc with PAH may be asymptomatic, particularly if early in the disease or if the patient is sedentary. When symptomatic, the primary clinical manifestation is exertional dyspnea, which results from the inability to adequately increase cardiac output during exercise. Lethargy and fatigue may also be present in early stages, whereas syncope, chest pain, edema, or symptoms at rest emerge only in very advanced cases when PAH progresses and causes right heart failure.[39,40] Less common symptoms include cough, hemoptysis, and hoarseness caused by compression of the left recurrent laryngeal nerve by a dilated main pulmonary artery. At physical examination, patients may present with jugular venous distension, hepatomegaly, peripheral edema, ascites, or cool extremities. At auscultation, a pronounced pulmonary component of the second heart sound, a pansystolic murmur of tricuspid regurgitation, a diastolic murmur of pulmonary insufficiency, or a right ventricular fourth sound may be heard.[39]

Monitoring and Screening for Pulmonary Arterial Hypertension in Systemic Sclerosis

Given the high prevalence and poor survival of SSc-PAH, and that aggressive management of mild disease may be associated with better outcomes,[2,41] screening is critical. Although screening programs can identify patients in early stages,[42] further studies are needed to validate these algorithms. Current European Society of Cardiology (ESC)/European Respiratory Society (ERS) guidelines[43] recommend yearly echocardiographic screening in asymptomatic patients with SSc (evidence class I, level B).[39] Updated consensus and evidence-based recommendations for screening and early detection of CTD-PAH[44] recommend annual screening of all patients with SSc for PAH using at least PFTs with DLCO, and echocardiogram, and to refer for further evaluation with RHC if studies are suggestive of PAH (**Box 2**).

ItinerAIR screening algorithm

Proposed by a multidisciplinary board of experts in France, the ItinerAIR algorithm is intended to identify patients with SSc at high risk for PAH by considering the peak

---

Box 2
General recommendations, initial screening evaluation, and frequency of noninvasive tests for early detection of CTD-associated PAH

General recommendations

   All patients with SSc should be screened for PAH (moderate)

   Patients with MCTD or other CTDs with scleroderma features (scleroderma spectrum disorders) should be screened in a similar manner to patients with SSc (very low)

   Screening is not recommended for asymptomatic patients with MCTD or other CTDs (including SLE, rheumatoid arthritis, inflammatory myositis, Sjögren syndrome) without features of scleroderma (low to moderate)

   For unexplained signs and symptoms of PH in patients with MCTD, SLE, or other CTDs without scleroderma features, consider the diagnostic algorithm evaluation for PH (moderate)

   All patients with SSc and scleroderma spectrum disorders with positive results on a noninvasive screen (discussed later) should be referred for RHC (high)

   RHC is mandatory for diagnosis of PAH (high)

   Acute vasodilator testing is not required as part of the evaluation of PAH in patients with SSc, scleroderma spectrum disorders, or other CTDs (moderate to high)

Initial screening evaluation

   PFTs with DLCO (high)

   Transthoracic echocardiogram (high)

   NT-proBNP (moderate)

   DETECT algorithm if DLCO less than 60% of predicted and disease duration greater than 3 years (moderate)

Frequency of noninvasive tests

   Transthoracic echocardiogram annually as a screening test (low)

   Transthoracic echocardiogram if new signs or symptoms develop (high)

   PFTs with DLCO annually as a screening test (low)

   PFTs with DLCO if new signs or symptoms develop (low)

   NT-proBNP if new signs or symptoms develop (low)

The quality of evidence, which was assessed according to the Grading of Recommendations Assessment, Development and Evaluation Working Group, is shown in parentheses at the end of each statement.
Abbreviations: DETECT, Detection of PAH in SSc; DLCO, diffusing capacity for carbon monoxide; MCTD, mixed connective tissue disease; NT-proBNP, N-terminal pro–brain natriuretic peptide; SLE, systemic lupus erythematosus.
From Khanna D, Gladue H, Channick R, et al. Recommendations for screening and detection of connective tissue disease-associated pulmonary arterial hypertension. Arthritis Rheum 2013;65(12):3196; with permission.

velocity of tricuspid regurgitation (VTR) on echocardiogram. High-risk patients, defined by a VTR greater than 3 m/s or a VTR between 2.5 and 3 m/s with dyspnea not explained by another cause, undergo RHC to confirm the diagnosis.[45] This approach allowed early detection of PAH in 55% and postcapillary PH in a further 10% of the high-risk patients.[13] In order to decrease the false-positive rate (36%), the previous algorithm was revised, and patients with a VTR greater than 2.8 m/s with unexplained dyspnea or a VTR greater than 3 m/s were considered high risk (false-positive rate with this approach decreased to 30.7%).[14]

Australian algorithm
N-terminal pro–brain natriuretic peptide (NT-proBNP) has been shown in several studies to be predictive of the presence of PAH[45,46] or its future[34,46,47] development in patients with SSc. In an Australian cohort of patients with SSc, an algorithm was developed in which patients screened positive if NT-proBNP was greater than or equal to 209.8 pg/mL, and/or DLCO was less than 70.3% with FVC%/DLCO% greater than or equal to 1.82. This approach showed a sensitivity of 100% and specificity of 77.8% for detecting PAH in a retrospective cohort, but it has not been validated prospectively.[48]

Detection of pulmonary arterial hypertension in systemic sclerosis algorithm
Recently, a 2-step algorithm, called the DETECT (Detection of PAH in SSc) algorithm, was developed based on 1 prospective international multicenter study of 466 patients with SSc considered at high risk for PAH, with disease duration of at least 3 years, and a DLCO less than 60% of predicted. Step 1 uses 6 simple assessments (FVC percent predicted/DLCO percent predicted, current/past telangiectasias, serum ACA, serum NT-proBNP, serum urate, and right axis deviation on electrocardiogram) to determine continued evaluation with echocardiography. Step 2 uses the step 1 score and 2 echocardiographic measures (right atrium area and VTR) to determine whether the patient should undergo RHC. Because reporting parameters are variable between centers, physicians should specifically ask for right atrium area and VTR from the echocardiographer. Although it needs to be validated in a prospective cohort, this noninvasive algorithm has a high sensitivity (96%) and minimizes missed diagnoses compared with ESC/ERS guidelines.[39,43] The DETECT algorithm has been included in updated recommendations for screening and early detection of PAH in patients with SSc (see **Box 2**).[44]

Diagnostic Approach for Pulmonary Arterial Hypertension
The diagnosis of PAH is often delayed or missed because symptoms usually overlap with other SSc manifestations.[49] RHC is the gold standard for the definitive diagnosis of PAH, but, given its invasive nature, it is only recommended in those patients with high probability of PAH based on screening evaluations.[13] The diagnosis of PAH is defined by mPAP greater than or equal to 25 mm Hg at rest, and PAWP less than or equal to 15 mm Hg (to exclude PH secondary to left heart disease). Increased pulmonary vascular resistance (PVR) and TPG also support the diagnosis. In addition, vasoreactivity testing with adenosine, nitric oxide, or prostacyclin may be performed, but because patients with SSc-PAH are rarely responders,[50] most recent guidelines do not routinely recommend this test in SSc.[51] RHC is the confirmatory diagnostic study for PAH, but several studies should be done before and/or in conjunction with RHC to exclude other causes of PH, and to determine PH severity and prognosis.

PFTs are reliable, easily interpretable, and inexpensive tools[50] that are included in screening algorithms, allow identification of underlying pulmonary disease contributing to PH, and are helpful in determining disease severity and prognosis.[2] Patients with SSc with PAH almost always have decreased DLCO in the range of 40% to 70% of predicted.[39] A decreased total lung capacity, decreased FVC, and a normal or increased forced expiratory volume in 1 second/FVC ratio may indicate the presence and severity of ILD.[39]

The 6-minute walk test is used to identify and monitor hypoxemia and exercise intolerance, and is the primary outcome measure used in most clinical trials for PAH-specific medications. A forehead rather than finger probe should be used to obtain reliable oximetry measures given the poor distal blood flow of patients with SSc.[52] The 6-minute walk distance (6MWD) is not specific or sensitive for PAH in patients with SSc because it can also be abnormal because of ILD, anemia, arthritis, or muscle disease.[50] However, the 6MWD correlates with hemodynamics and is useful for monitoring progression of disease, with a minimal clinically important difference, defined as a change of 33 m in a cohort of patients with PAH (24% CTD-PAH).[53]

In patients with advanced PAH, a typical electrocardiographic finding is right axis deviation of the QRS complex, which reflects right atrial dilatation and right ventricular hypertrophy.[50] One observational study of 36 patients with SSc found an abnormal 24-hour Holter monitoring study in more than half of the patients (predominantly ventricular ectopy and monomorphic tachycardias), and these patients were more likely to have PH by echocardiogram.[54,55] This finding has not been confirmed in larger studies.

High-resolution computed tomography (HRCT) is a necessary adjunctive test in the evaluation of patients with suspected PAH. A pulmonary artery diameter greater than 30 mm, right heart enlargement, or pericardial effusion/thickening are HRCT features that suggest PAH and should prompt more precise PAH assessments.[50] In addition, HRCT is the gold standard to diagnose and determine the extent of ILD or pulmonary fibrosis because many patients with PAH also have some underlying ILD. The HRCT can be helpful in differentiating World Health Organization (WHO) group 1 from group 3 PH in that the latter group by definition has severe pulmonary fibrosis. In addition, HRCT findings, including lymph node enlargement, centrilobular ground-glass opacities, and septal lines, can suggest the presence of PVOD.[56]

TTE is a useful noninvasive tool for screening for PAH, exclusion of left-sided heart disease, and monitoring severity and progression of disease. It provides an estimated pulmonary arterial pressure (PAP) based on the peak velocity of the jet of tricuspid regurgitation (VTR), but a particular cutoff value cannot confirm the diagnosis.[39] Although sensitivity is low, it has been shown to have a high specificity, high positive predictive value, and large area under the curve in identifying SSc-PAH.[57] Left-sided systolic or diastolic dysfunction can also be evaluated. The severity of PH can be assessed with TTE by identifying the presence of right atrial and/or ventricular enlargement, right ventricular (RV) dysfunction, and/or a large pericardial effusion. In addition, novel echocardiographic parameters are useful in determining severity and prognosis in SSc-PAH. For example, the tricuspid annular plane systolic excursion, a measurement in centimeters of the total systolic displacement of the tricuspid annulus toward the RV apex, which estimates RV function, has been shown to correlate with hemodynamics and survival in patients with SSc-PAH. A value of less than or equal to 1.7 cm confers an almost 4-fold increased risk of death (HR, 3.81; 95% CI, 1.31–11.1; $P<.01$).[58] Other novel TTE measures of RV systolic performance, including tissue Doppler systolic velocity and fractional area change, have also been shown to correlate negatively with PVR in patients with SSc-PAH.[59]

INTERSTITIAL LUNG DISEASE AND PULMONARY HYPERTENSION IN SYSTEMIC SCLEROSIS

Although PAH is the most common form of PH in SSc, some patients develop respiratory disease–associated PH (group 3). ILD-associated PH is diagnosed when PH presents in a patient who has extensive ILD, and alternative causes of PH are excluded. One retrospective dual-center study of 70 patients with SSc with ILD-associated PH showed that these patients have an extremely poor prognosis, with 1-year, 2-year, and 3-year survival rates of 71%, 39%, and 21%, respectively. Furthermore, the risk of death was higher for patients with worsening oxygenation and reduced renal function, and PAH therapies did not show clear benefits after a mean of 7.7 ± 6.2 months of treatment.[60] A multicenter UK study of 429 patients with CTD-PH (73% SSc-PH) showed that the group with respiratory-associated PH had a lower gas transfer (TL_{CO}), poorer exercise tolerance, and worse survival compared with patients with SSc-PAH.[41,61] In a multicenter European study of 83 patients with SSc with confirmed PH by RHC, 22 patients had PH secondary to ILD. These patients were more likely to be men (odds ratio [OR], 4.7; 95% CI, 1.7–12.5; $P = .003$), and to have diffuse cutaneous SSc (OR, 13.1; 95% CI, 2.9–59.1; $P = .0008$).[16]

Exercise-induced Pulmonary Arterial Hypertension

Exercise-induced PAH is no longer part of the classification criteria for PAH,[5,6] but exercise can likely unmask PAH in high-risk patients with SSc. One study of 54 patients with SSc showed that 44% of patients had a positive exercise echocardiogram, defined by an increase in RVSP of at least 20 mm Hg with exercise. PAH was confirmed by RHC in 81% of these patients.[35] A multicenter prospective study of 164 patients with SSc and normal resting pulmonary artery systolic pressure (PASP) (defined as <40 mm Hg) showed that 42% had a significant increase in PASP during exercise (defined as >50 mm Hg). Note that PASP increase was associated with PVR increase in only 5% of patients, suggesting heterogeneous mechanisms causing exercise-induced PAH.[62] One retrospective cohort study of 19 patients with SSc evaluated the performance of a noninvasive stress test (step test) in identifying PAH. Investigators estimated a sensitivity of 100%, specificity of 75%, positive predictive value of 94%, and negative predictive value of 100% for this step test using a cutoff of 4 mm Hg in change of end-tidal carbon dioxide (ΔP_{ETCO2}) for defining a positive test. In addition, ΔP_{ETCO2} was inversely correlated with mPAP on RHC ($r = -0.82$; $P<.0001$), whereas correlations with PASP on TTE ($r = 0.74$; $P = .0004$), and FVC/DLCO were lower ($r = 0.53$; $P = .034$).[63] Condliffe and colleagues[41] showed that survival of patients with SSc-PAH with exercise was better compared with patients with PAH at rest, but a significant proportion had evidence of disease progression. Identifying patients with exercise-induced PAH may be a sensitive way to detect early PAH and improve outcomes with early treatment.

Predictors of Mortality in Systemic Sclerosis–Pulmonary Arterial Hypertension

The development of PAH in patients with SSc has a major impact on survival. Although some studies have shown that mortality has decreased in the current treatment era,[64] PAH is still one of the leading causes of death,[65] and increases the risk of death by 3-fold compared with patients with SSc without PAH.[66] Furthermore, patients with SSc-PAH have a higher mortality than patients with IPAH,[13] and other causes of CTD-PAH.[67] From the registry to evaluate early and long-term PAH disease management (REVEAL) registry, a US multicenter, observational registry of patients with RHC-confirmed PAH, the 1-year and 3-year survival rates for newly diagnosed SSc-PAH were 78% and 54% respectively.[68] One meta-analysis of 22 studies and 2244 patients with SSc-PAH determined pooled 1-year, 2-year, and 3-year survival rates of 81%, 64%, and 52% respectively.[69] Better outcomes (1-year, 2-year, and 3-year cumulative survival rates of 93%, 88%, and 75%, respectively) were found in the US PHAROS registry consisting of 131 patients with SSc with incident PAH and mild disease followed over a mean of 2 ± 1.4 years.[2] In this same study, age more than 60 years, male gender, functional class IV status, and DLCO less than 39% of predicted were the strongest predictors of mortality.[2] In the REVEAL registry, in addition to age and male gender, the following were also significant predictors of mortality in patients with SSc-PAH: low baseline systolic blood pressure, poor exercise capacity, increased mean right atrial pressure, and increased PVR.[70] As mentioned earlier, NT-proBNP is highly relevant for screening and diagnosis, and has been shown to be a predictor of mortality in some cohorts.[71] A 10-fold increase in NT-proBNP levels has been associated with a 3-fold increased risk of death in a UK cohort.[46]

Novel Biomarkers

A recent proteome-wide analysis showed that levels of CXC chemokine ligand 4 (CXCL4), a chemokine with antiangiogenic and profibrotic properties, were increased in patients with SSc and correlated with the presence and progression of PAH.[72] Other cytokines, such as tumor necrosis factor-alpha, interleukin (IL) 1-beta, intracellular adhesion molecule 1 (ICAM-1), and IL-6, and markers of vascular injury such as vascular cell adhesion molecule 1 (VCAM-1), vascular endothelial growth factor, and von Willebrand factor (vWF) have also been found to be increased in patients with SSc-PAH.[52] Furthermore, vWF has been associated with PAP greater than 40 mm Hg and to predict the future development of PAH.[73,74] In addition, one study showed that patients from the PHAROS registry with incident SSc-PAH expressed higher levels of hepatocyte grown factor than patients with SSc without definite PAH. These levels also correlated with increased RVSP on echocardiogram.[75] In addition, a small study of 20 patients with SSc-PAH found higher serum levels of endoglin, and endothelin-1 (ET-1) compared with healthy controls, suggesting a potential role as PAH biomarkers.[76,77]

Treatment

Modern treatment of PAH has resulted in significant improvement in survival; however, patients with idiopathic PAH consistently have better outcomes than patients with SSc-PAH. Screening patients with SSc could allow early identification of PAH,[78] followed by aggressive initiation and escalation of therapy, with the goal of improving prognosis.[79] Potential factors contributing to the poor outcomes in SSc-PAH include older age, presence of comorbidities, and multisystem internal organ involvement, including cardiac, renal, parenchymal lung, and/or gastrointestinal disease. In addition, these patients are more likely to have venule involvement including PVOD. Once a diagnosis of PAH is confirmed by RHC, treatment with PAH-specific therapies should be considered (**Fig. 1**). Most of these drugs have not been specifically studied in SSc-PAH. High-dose calcium channel blockers are not usually indicated for patients with SSc-PAH because a low percentage of patients have shown long-term response. In addition, current guidelines recommend that, if patients have an inadequate response to monotherapy with a particular PAH-specific medication, combination therapy should be initiated. The choice of therapy should consider the severity of functional limitation, comorbidities, and patient preference.

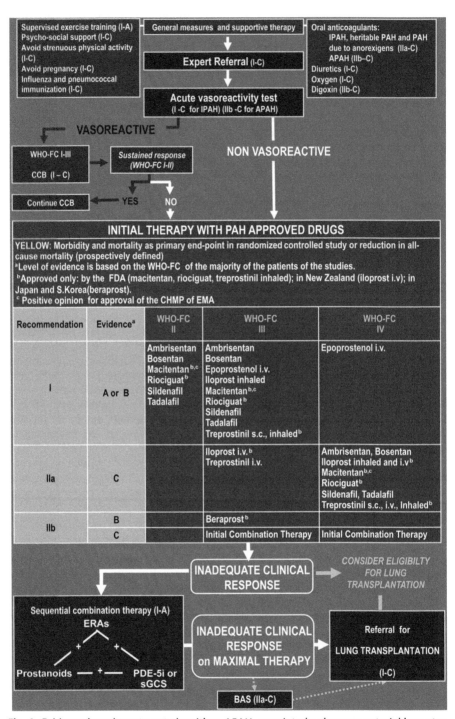

Fig. 1. Evidence-based treatment algorithm. APAH, associated pulmonary arterial hypertension; BAS, balloon atrial septostomy; CCB, calcium channel blockers; ERA, endothelin receptor antagonist; FC, functional class; IPAH, idiopathic pulmonary arterial hypertension; i.v., intravenous; PDE-5i, phosphodiesterase type-5 inhibitor; s.c., subcutaneous; sGCS, soluble guanylate cyclase stimulators; WHO-FC, World Health Organization functional class. (*From* Galie N, Corris PA, Frost A, et al. Updated treatment algorithm of pulmonary arterial hypertension. J Am Coll Cardiol 2013;62(25 Suppl):D63; with permission.)

Supportive therapies

Patients with hypoxemia at rest (arterial blood oxygen pressure <60 mm Hg or arterial oxygen saturation <90%) or with activity should receive supplemental oxygen. Diuretics should be given to patients with fluid retention secondary to right heart failure. There is conflicting evidence regarding the role of anticoagulation in SSc-PAH.[80] One Australian observational study concluded that there is a low probability that warfarin improves survival in SSc-PAH.[81] Given this evidence and the risk for gastrointestinal bleeding, its use should be considered only on a case-by-case basis, and perhaps in patients with antiphospholipid antibodies.

Prostanoids

The first class of agents that was approved for the treatment of PAH is prostanoids, which are potent pulmonary and systemic vasodilators that stimulate cyclic AMP. Prostanoids have been shown in clinical trials to improve symptoms, functional capacity, and hemodynamic parameters in patients with SSc-PAH. Administered as a continuous intravenous infusion, epoprostenol has resulted in improved hemodynamics and functional class, as well as better survival rates in patients with SSc-PAH.[82,83] Treprostinil is available in subcutaneous,[84] intravenous,[85] inhaled,[86] and oral formulations,[87,88] because of improvements in exercise capacity, functional class, and hemodynamics in PAH clinical trials that included patients with SSc-PAH. Iloprost is also available in inhaled formulations.[89,90]

Endothelin receptor antagonists

Endothelin receptor antagonists (ETRA) are oral agents that block the interaction of ET-1 with its receptors (ET_A and ET_B), interfering with its vasoconstrictive effects. Bosentan, the first dual receptor blocker to receive regulatory approval, has been shown to increase 6MWD, to delay clinical progression,[91,92] and to improve survival in SSc-PAH.[57] Macitentan, a recently approved dual receptor blocker, has been shown to improve morbidity and mortality in patients with PAH.[93,94] Data evaluating its efficacy and safety specifically in SSc-PAH are limited. Ambrisentan, the only currently approved ET_A-specific ETRA, has shown modest benefits in 2 multicenter randomized trials including patients with SSc-PAH.[95]

Phosphodiesterase-5 inhibitors and soluble guanylate cyclase stimulator

By inhibiting the hydrolysis of cyclic GMP, phosphodiesterase-5 inhibitors are oral agents that increase the concentration of nitric oxide, with consequent vasodilatory, antiproliferative, and proapoptotic effects that may reverse pulmonary artery remodeling. In a subgroup analysis of patients with SSc-PAH, 20 mg 3 times daily of sildenafil showed an improvement in 6MWD, and decrease in functional class, pulmonary artery pressure, and PVR.[96] Although a separate SSc analysis has not been done, tadalafil is effective in PAH treatment, including CTD-PAH.[97]

Riociguat is a novel soluble guanylate cyclase stimulator that is effective for the treatment of PAH.[98] The phase 3, double-blind study of 443 patients with symptomatic PAH included 111 patients with CTD-PAH. Patients were assigned to receive placebo, up to 1.5 mg 3 times daily, or up to 2.5 mg 3 times daily of riociguat. By week 12, the 6MWD increased by a mean of 30 m in the 2.5 mg–maximum group (in patients who were receiving ETRA, prostanoids, or no other treatment), whereas it decreased by a mean of 6 m in the placebo group.[98]

Transplant

Lung transplantation remains an option for appropriate candidates with severe symptoms despite treatment with intravenous prostanoids, either alone or in combination with other drugs. One observational study of 29 patients with SSc, 70 patients with idiopathic pulmonary fibrosis, and 38 patients with IPAH concluded that the 2-year survival after lung transplantation was similar among the groups (61%, 64%, and 63% respectively).[99] A systematic review of 7 observational studies evaluating post-transplant survival concluded that patients with SSc-PAH had 1-year, 2-year, and 3-year survival rates of 59% to 93%, 49% to 80%, and 46% to 79%, respectively, which was similar to survival of patients with IPAH and idiopathic pulmonary fibrosis requiring lung transplantation.[100] A recent retrospective nationwide study of 3763 adults who underwent lung transplantation in the United States between 2005 and 2012 concluded that a diagnosis of SSc was associated with a 48% relative increase in the 1-year mortality compared with a diagnosis of ILD not associated with SSc, but had no increase in risk of death at 1 year compared with PAH not caused by SSc.[101]

FUTURE CONSIDERATIONS/SUMMARY

PAH is an important and fatal complication in patients with SSc. Identifying patients who are at high risk and confirming the diagnosis early with RHC may allow aggressive initiation and escalation of therapy that could potentially improve prognosis. However, clinical outcomes are still not as good as those of patients with IPAH making early diagnosis and aggressive treatment imperative. Several algorithms and consensus-based recommendations are available for screening. RHC is the gold standard for the definitive diagnosis of PAH, and should be performed in those patients in whom this diagnosis is suspected. For suitable patients with severe disease despite adequate vasodilator therapy, lung transplantation is a reasonable option.

REFERENCES

1. Mukerjee D, St George D, Coleiro B, et al. Prevalence and outcome in systemic sclerosis associated pulmonary arterial hypertension: application of a registry approach. Ann Rheum Dis 2003;62(11):1088–93.
2. Chung L, Domsic RT, Lingala B, et al. Survival and predictors of mortality in systemic sclerosis-associated pulmonary arterial hypertension: outcomes from the pulmonary hypertension assessment and recognition of outcomes in scleroderma registry. Arthritis Care Res 2014;66(3):489–95.
3. Launay D, Sitbon O, Hachulla E, et al. Survival in systemic sclerosis-associated pulmonary arterial hypertension in the modern management era. Ann Rheum Dis 2013;72(12):1940–6.
4. Badesch DB, Champion HC, Sanchez MA, et al. Diagnosis and assessment of pulmonary arterial hypertension. J Am Coll Cardiol 2009;54(1 Suppl):S55–66.
5. Simonneau G, Robbins IM, Beghetti M, et al. Updated clinical classification of pulmonary hypertension. J Am Coll Cardiol 2009;54(1 Suppl):S43–54.
6. Simonneau G, Gatzoulis MA, Adatia I, et al. Updated clinical classification of pulmonary hypertension. J Am Coll Cardiol 2013;62(25 Suppl):D34–41.
7. Domsic RT, Chung L, Gomberg-Maitland M, et al. Pulmonary hypertension assessment and recognition of outcomes in scleroderma (PHAROS): comparison of outcomes in subtypes of pulmonary hypertension. Arthritis Rheum 2010;62(10S):S245.
8. Johnson SR, Patsios D, Hwang DM, et al. Pulmonary veno-occlusive disease and scleroderma associated pulmonary hypertension. J Rheumatol 2006; 33(11):2347–50.
9. McGuire F, Kennelly T, Tillack T, et al. Pulmonary capillary hemangiomatosis associated with CREST syndrome: a case report and review of the literature. Respiration 2010;80(5):435–8.

10. Montani D, Price LC, Dorfmuller P, et al. Pulmonary veno-occlusive disease. Eur Respir J 2009;33(1):189–200.
11. Montani D, Achouh L, Dorfmuller P, et al. Pulmonary veno-occlusive disease: clinical, functional, radiologic, and hemodynamic characteristics and outcome of 24 cases confirmed by histology. Medicine 2008;87(4):220–33.
12. O'Callaghan DS, Dorfmuller P, Jais X, et al. Pulmonary veno-occlusive disease: the bete noire of pulmonary hypertension in connective tissue diseases? Presse Med 2011;40(1 Pt 2):e65–78.
13. Hachulla E, Gressin V, Guillevin L, et al. Early detection of pulmonary arterial hypertension in systemic sclerosis: a French nationwide prospective multicenter study. Arthritis Rheum 2005;52(12):3792–800.
14. Hachulla E, de Groote P, Gressin V, et al. The three-year incidence of pulmonary arterial hypertension associated with systemic sclerosis in a multicenter nationwide longitudinal study in France. Arthritis Rheum 2009;60(6):1831–9.
15. Hsu VM, Chung L, Hummers LK, et al. Development of pulmonary hypertension in a high-risk population with systemic sclerosis in the Pulmonary Hypertension Assessment and Recognition of Outcomes in Scleroderma (PHAROS) cohort study. Semin Arthritis Rheum 2014;44(1):55–62.
16. Avouac J, Airo P, Meune C, et al. Prevalence of pulmonary hypertension in systemic sclerosis in European Caucasians and metaanalysis of 5 studies. J Rheumatol 2010;37(11):2290–8.
17. Schachna L, Wigley FM, Chang B, et al. Age and risk of pulmonary arterial hypertension in scleroderma. Chest 2003;124(6):2098–104.
18. Scorza R, Caronni M, Bazzi S, et al. Post-menopause is the main risk factor for developing isolated pulmonary hypertension in systemic sclerosis. Ann N Y Acad Sci 2002;966:238–46.
19. Beretta L, Caronni M, Origgi L, et al. Hormone replacement therapy may prevent the development of isolated pulmonary hypertension in patients with systemic sclerosis and limited cutaneous involvement. Scand J Rheumatol 2006;35(6):468–71.
20. Cox SR, Walker JG, Coleman M, et al. Isolated pulmonary hypertension in scleroderma. Intern Med J 2005;35(1):28–33.
21. Hachulla E, Launay D, Mouthon L, et al. Is pulmonary arterial hypertension really a late complication of systemic sclerosis? Chest 2009;136(5):1211–9.
22. Shah AA, Wigley FM, Hummers LK. Telangiectases in scleroderma: a potential clinical marker of pulmonary arterial hypertension. J Rheumatol 2010;37(1):98–104.
23. Steen VD. Autoantibodies in systemic sclerosis. Semin Arthritis Rheum 2005; 35(1):35–42.
24. Kampolis C, Plastiras S, Vlachoyiannopoulos P, et al. The presence of anticentromere antibodies may predict progression of estimated pulmonary arterial systolic pressure in systemic sclerosis. Scand J Rheumatol 2008;37(4):278–83.
25. Aggarwal R, Lucas M, Fertig N, et al. Anti-U3 RNP autoantibodies in systemic sclerosis. Arthritis Rheum 2009;60(4):1112–8.
26. Steen VD, Lucas M, Fertig N, et al. Pulmonary arterial hypertension and severe pulmonary fibrosis in systemic sclerosis patients with a nucleolar antibody. J Rheumatol 2007;34(11):2230–5.
27. Assous N, Allanore Y, Batteux F, et al. Prevalence of antiphospholipid antibodies in systemic sclerosis and association with primitive pulmonary arterial hypertension and endothelial injury. Clin Exp Rheumatol 2005;23(2):199–204.
28. Steen V, Medsger TA Jr. Predictors of isolated pulmonary hypertension in patients with systemic sclerosis and limited cutaneous involvement. Arthritis Rheum 2003;48(2):516–22.

29. Yaqub A, Chung L. Epidemiology and risk factors for pulmonary hypertension in systemic sclerosis. Curr Rheumatol Rep 2013;15(1):302.

30. Dib H, Tamby MC, Bussone G, et al. Targets of anti-endothelial cell antibodies in pulmonary hypertension and scleroderma. Eur Respir J 2012;39(6):1405–14.

31. Negi VS, Tripathy NK, Misra R, et al. Antiendothelial cell antibodies in scleroderma correlate with severe digital ischemia and pulmonary arterial hypertension. J Rheumatol 1998;25(3):462–6.

32. Becker MO, Kill A, Kutsche M, et al. Vascular receptor autoantibodies in pulmonary arterial hypertension associated with systemic sclerosis. Am J Respir Crit Care Med 2014;190(7):808–17.

33. Steen VD, Graham G, Conte C, et al. Isolated diffusing capacity reduction in systemic sclerosis. Arthritis Rheum 1992;35(7):765–70.

34. Allanore Y, Borderie D, Avouac J, et al. High N-terminal pro-brain natriuretic peptide levels and low diffusing capacity for carbon monoxide as independent predictors of the occurrence of precapillary pulmonary arterial hypertension in patients with systemic sclerosis. Arthritis Rheum 2008;58(1):284–91.

35. Steen V, Chou M, Shanmugam V, et al. Exercise-induced pulmonary arterial hypertension in patients with systemic sclerosis. Chest 2008;134(1):146–51.

36. Shah AA, Chung SE, Wigley FM, et al. Changes in estimated right ventricular systolic pressure predict mortality and pulmonary hypertension in a cohort of scleroderma patients. Ann Rheum Dis 2013;72(7):1136–40.

37. Valerio CJ, Schreiber BE, Handler CE, et al. Borderline mean pulmonary artery pressure in patients with systemic sclerosis: transpulmonary gradient predicts risk of developing pulmonary hypertension. Arthritis Rheum 2013;65(4):1074–84.

38. Bae S, Saggar R, Bolster MB, et al. Baseline characteristics and follow-up in patients with normal haemodynamics versus borderline mean pulmonary arterial pressure in systemic sclerosis: results from the PHAROS registry. Ann Rheum Dis 2012;71(8):1335–42.

39. Galie N, Hoeper MM, Humbert M, et al. Guidelines for the diagnosis and treatment of pulmonary hypertension. Eur Respir J 2009;34(6):1219–63.

40. Saukkonen K, Tan TC, Sharma A, et al. Case 9-2014: a 34-year-old woman with increasing dyspnea (case records of the Massachusetts General Hospital). N Engl J Med 2014;370(12):1149–57.

41. Condliffe R, Kiely DG, Peacock AJ, et al. Connective tissue disease-associated pulmonary arterial hypertension in the modern treatment era. Am J Respir Crit Care Med 2009;179(2):151–7.

42. Humbert M, Yaici A, de Groote P, et al. Screening for pulmonary arterial hypertension in patients with systemic sclerosis: clinical characteristics at diagnosis and long-term survival. Arthritis Rheum 2011;63(11):3522–30.

43. Coghlan JG, Denton CP, Grunig E, et al. Evidence-based detection of pulmonary arterial hypertension in systemic sclerosis: the DETECT study. Ann Rheum Dis 2014;73(7):1340–9.

44. Khanna D, Gladue H, Channick R, et al. Recommendations for screening and detection of connective tissue disease-associated pulmonary arterial hypertension. Arthritis Rheum 2013;65(12):3194–201.

45. Hachulla E, Gressin V, Guillevin L, et al. Pulmonary arterial hypertension in systemic sclerosis: definition of a screening algorithm for early detection (the ItinerAIR-Sclerodermie Study). Rev Med Interne 2004;25(5):340–7 [in French].

46. Williams MH, Handler CE, Akram R, et al. Role of N-terminal brain natriuretic peptide (N-TproBNP) in scleroderma-associated pulmonary arterial hypertension. Eur Heart J 2006;27(12):1485–94.

47. Cavagna L, Caporali R, Klersy C, et al. Comparison of brain natriuretic peptide (BNP) and NT-proBNP in screening for pulmonary arterial hypertension in patients with systemic sclerosis. J Rheumatol 2010;37(10):2064–70.
48. Thakkar V, Stevens WM, Prior D, et al. N-terminal pro-brain natriuretic peptide in a novel screening algorithm for pulmonary arterial hypertension in systemic sclerosis: a case-control study. Arthritis Res Ther 2012;14(3):R143.
49. Gladue H, Steen V, Allanore Y, et al. Combination of echocardiographic and pulmonary function test measures improves sensitivity for diagnosis of systemic sclerosis-associated pulmonary arterial hypertension: analysis of 2 cohorts. J Rheumatol 2013;40(10):1706–11.
50. Fischer A, Bull TM, Steen VD. Practical approach to screening for scleroderma-associated pulmonary arterial hypertension. Arthritis Care Res 2012;64(3):303–10.
51. Hoeper MM, Bogaard HJ, Condliffe R, et al. Definitions and diagnosis of pulmonary hypertension. J Am Coll Cardiol 2013;62(25 Suppl):D42–50.
52. Wilsher M, Good N, Hopkins R, et al. The six-minute walk test using forehead oximetry is reliable in the assessment of scleroderma lung disease. Respirology 2012;17(4):647–52.
53. Mathai SC, Puhan MA, Lam D, et al. The minimal important difference in the 6-minute walk test for patients with pulmonary arterial hypertension. Am J Respir Crit Care Med 2012;186(5):428–33.
54. Tzelepis GE, Kelekis NL, Plastiras SC, et al. Pattern and distribution of myocardial fibrosis in systemic sclerosis: a delayed enhanced magnetic resonance imaging study. Arthritis Rheum 2007;56(11):3827–36.
55. Vacca A, Meune C, Gordon J, et al. Cardiac arrhythmias and conduction defects in systemic sclerosis. Rheumatology (Oxford) 2014;53(7):1172–7.
56. Gunther S, Jais X, Maitre S, et al. Computed tomography findings of pulmonary venoocclusive disease in scleroderma patients presenting with precapillary pulmonary hypertension. Arthritis Rheum 2012;64(9):2995–3005.
57. Hsu VM, Moreyra AE, Wilson AC, et al. Assessment of pulmonary arterial hypertension in patients with systemic sclerosis: comparison of noninvasive tests with results of right-heart catheterization. J Rheumatol 2008;35(3):458–65.
58. Mathai SC, Sibley CT, Forfia PR, et al. Tricuspid annular plane systolic excursion is a robust outcome measure in systemic sclerosis-associated pulmonary arterial hypertension. J Rheumatol 2011;38(11):2410–8.
59. Gopal DM, Doldt B, Finch K, et al. Relation of novel echocardiographic measures to invasive hemodynamic assessment in scleroderma-associated pulmonary arterial hypertension. Arthritis Care Res 2014;66(9):1386–94.
60. Le Pavec J, Girgis RE, Lechtzin N, et al. Systemic sclerosis-related pulmonary hypertension associated with interstitial lung disease: impact of pulmonary arterial hypertension therapies. Arthritis Rheum 2011;63(8):2456–64.
61. Mathai SC, Hummers LK, Champion HC, et al. Survival in pulmonary hypertension associated with the scleroderma spectrum of diseases: impact of interstitial lung disease. Arthritis Rheum 2009;60(2):569–77.
62. Gargani L, Pignone A, Agoston G, et al. Clinical and echocardiographic correlations of exercise-induced pulmonary hypertension in systemic sclerosis: a multicenter study. Am Heart J 2013;165(2):200–7.
63. Bernstein EJ, Mandl LA, Gordon JK, et al. Submaximal heart and pulmonary evaluation: a novel noninvasive test to identify pulmonary hypertension in patients with systemic sclerosis. Arthritis Care Res 2013;65(10):1713–8.

64. Williams MH, Das C, Handler CE, et al. Systemic sclerosis associated pulmonary hypertension: improved survival in the current era. Heart 2006;92(7): 926–32.

65. Tyndall AJ, Bannert B, Vonk M, et al. Causes and risk factors for death in systemic sclerosis: a study from the EULAR Scleroderma Trials and Research (EUSTAR) database. Ann Rheum Dis 2010;69(10):1809–15.

66. Hesselstrand R, Wildt M, Ekmehag B, et al. Survival in patients with pulmonary arterial hypertension associated with systemic sclerosis from a Swedish single centre: prognosis still poor and prediction difficult. Scand J Rheumatol 2011; 40(2):127–32.

67. Chung L, Liu J, Parsons L, et al. Characterization of connective tissue disease-associated pulmonary arterial hypertension from REVEAL: identifying systemic sclerosis as a unique phenotype. Chest 2010;138(6):1383–94.

68. Chung L, Liu J, Parsons LS, et al. Response to 'survival in pulmonary hypertension registries: the importance of incident cases'. Chest 2011;139(6): 1548–9.

69. Lefevre G, Dauchet L, Hachulla E, et al. Survival and prognostic factors in systemic sclerosis-associated pulmonary hypertension: a systematic review and meta-analysis. Arthritis Rheum 2013;65(9):2412–23.

70. Chung L, Farber HW, Benza R, et al. Unique predictors of mortality in patients with pulmonary arterial hypertension associated with systemic sclerosis in the REVEAL registry. Chest 2014;146(6):1494–504.

71. Schioppo T, Artusi C, Ciavarella T, et al. N-TproBNP as biomarker in systemic sclerosis. Clin Rev Allergy Immunol 2012;43(3):292–301.

72. van Bon L, Affandi AJ, Broen J, et al. Proteome-wide analysis and CXCL4 as a biomarker in systemic sclerosis. N Engl J Med 2014;370(5):433–43.

73. Pendergrass SA, Hayes E, Farina G, et al. Limited systemic sclerosis patients with pulmonary arterial hypertension show biomarkers of inflammation and vascular injury. PLoS One 2010;5(8):e12106.

74. Barnes T, Gliddon A, Dore CJ, et al. Baseline vWF factor predicts the development of elevated pulmonary artery pressure in systemic sclerosis. Rheumatology (Oxford) 2012;51(9):1606–9.

75. Chung L, Cramb C, Robinson W, et al. Differential expression of hepatocyte growth factor (HGF) in patients with systemic sclerosis-associated pulmonary arterial hypertension. Arthritis Rheum 2012;64(10):S632.

76. Dimitroulas T, Giannakoulas G, Karvounis H, et al. Biomarkers in systemic sclerosis-related pulmonary arterial hypertension. Curr Vasc Pharmacol 2011; 9(2):213–9.

77. Coral-Alvarado P, Quintana G, Garces MF, et al. Potential biomarkers for detecting pulmonary arterial hypertension in patients with systemic sclerosis. Rheumatol Int 2009;29(9):1017–24.

78. Hassoun PM. Therapies for scleroderma-related pulmonary arterial hypertension. Expert Rev Respir Med 2009;3(2):187–96.

79. Taichman DB, Ornelas J, Chung L, et al. Pharmacologic therapy for pulmonary arterial hypertension in adults: CHEST guideline and expert panel report. Chest 2014;146(2):449–75.

80. Nikpour M, Stevens W, Proudman SM, et al. Should patients with systemic sclerosis-related pulmonary arterial hypertension be anticoagulated? Intern Med J 2013;43(5):599–603.

81. Johnson SR, Granton JT, Tomlinson GA, et al. Warfarin in systemic sclerosis-associated and idiopathic pulmonary arterial hypertension. A Bayesian

approach to evaluating treatment for uncommon disease. J Rheumatol 2012; 39(2):276–85.

82. Badesch DB, Tapson VF, McGoon MD, et al. Continuous intravenous epoprostenol for pulmonary hypertension due to the scleroderma spectrum of disease. A randomized, controlled trial. Ann Intern Med 2000;132(6):425–34.

83. Badesch DB, McGoon MD, Barst RJ, et al. Longterm survival among patients with scleroderma-associated pulmonary arterial hypertension treated with intravenous epoprostenol. J Rheumatol 2009;36(10):2244–9.

84. Oudiz RJ, Schilz RJ, Barst RJ, et al. Treprostinil, a prostacyclin analogue, in pulmonary arterial hypertension associated with connective tissue disease. Chest 2004;126(2):420–7.

85. Tapson VF, Gomberg-Maitland M, McLaughlin VV, et al. Safety and efficacy of IV treprostinil for pulmonary arterial hypertension: a prospective, multicenter, open-label, 12-week trial. Chest 2006;129(3):683–8.

86. McLaughlin VV, Benza RL, Rubin LJ, et al. Addition of inhaled treprostinil to oral therapy for pulmonary arterial hypertension: a randomized controlled clinical trial. J Am Coll Cardiol 2010;55(18):1915–22.

87. Tapson VF, Torres F, Kermeen F, et al. Oral treprostinil for the treatment of pulmonary arterial hypertension in patients on background endothelin receptor antagonist and/or phosphodiesterase type 5 inhibitor therapy (the FREEDOM-C study): a randomized controlled trial. Chest 2012;142(6):1383–90.

88. Jing ZC, Parikh K, Pulido T, et al. Efficacy and safety of oral treprostinil monotherapy for the treatment of pulmonary arterial hypertension: a randomized, controlled trial. Circulation 2013;127(5):624–33.

89. Olschewski H, Simonneau G, Galie N, et al. Inhaled iloprost for severe pulmonary hypertension. N Engl J Med 2002;347(5):322–9.

90. Caramaschi P, Volpe A, Tinazzi I, et al. Does cyclically iloprost infusion prevent severe isolated pulmonary hypertension in systemic sclerosis? Preliminary Results. Rheumatol Int 2006;27(2):203–5.

91. Rubin LJ, Badesch DB, Barst RJ, et al. Bosentan therapy for pulmonary arterial hypertension. N Engl J Med 2002;346(12):896–903.

92. Denton CP, Pope JE, Peter HH, et al. Long-term effects of bosentan on quality of life, survival, safety and tolerability in pulmonary arterial hypertension related to connective tissue diseases. Ann Rheum Dis 2008;67(9):1222–8.

93. Pulido T, Adzerikho I, Channick RN, et al. Macitentan and morbidity and mortality in pulmonary arterial hypertension. N Engl J Med 2013;369(9):809–18.

94. Macchia A, Mariani J, Tognoni G. Macitentan and pulmonary arterial hypertension. N Engl J Med 2014;370(1):82.

95. Galie N, Olschewski H, Oudiz RJ, et al. Ambrisentan for the treatment of pulmonary arterial hypertension: results of the ambrisentan in pulmonary arterial hypertension, randomized, double-blind, placebo-controlled, multicenter, efficacy (ARIES) study 1 and 2. Circulation 2008;117(23):3010–9.

96. Badesch DB, Hill NS, Burgess G, et al. Sildenafil for pulmonary arterial hypertension associated with connective tissue disease. J Rheumatol 2007;34(12):2417–22.

97. Galie N, Brundage BH, Ghofrani HA, et al. Tadalafil therapy for pulmonary arterial hypertension. Circulation 2009;119(22):2894–903.

98. Ghofrani HA, Galie N, Grimminger F, et al. Riociguat for the treatment of pulmonary arterial hypertension. N Engl J Med 2013;369(4):330–40.

99. Schachna L, Medsger TA Jr, Dauber JH, et al. Lung transplantation in scleroderma compared with idiopathic pulmonary fibrosis and idiopathic pulmonary arterial hypertension. Arthritis Rheum 2006;54(12):3954–61.

100. Khan IY, Singer LG, de Perrot M, et al. Survival after lung transplantation in systemic sclerosis. A systematic review. Respir Med 2013;107(12):2081–7.
101. Bernstein E, Peterson E, Bathon J, et al. One-year survival of adults with systemic sclerosis following lung transplantation: a nationwide cohort study. Arthritis Rheumatol 2014;66(11):S789.

Musculoskeletal Manifestations of Systemic Sclerosis

Kathleen B. Morrisroe, MBBS[a],
Mandana Nikpour, MBBS, FRACP, FRCPA, PhD[b,c,*],
Susanna M. Proudman, MBBS[d,e]

KEYWORDS

- Systemic sclerosis • Scleroderma • Musculoskeletal manifestations • Arthralgia
- Arthritis • Treatment • Rehabilitation

KEY POINTS

- Musculoskeletal (MSK) involvement in systemic sclerosis (SSc) occurs more frequently than expected, with a prevalence of 24% to 97%, and is associated with significant disability and psychosocial and economic burden.
- There is no formal classification system for MSK manifestations in SSc. MSK involvement presents as one or more of stiffness, arthritis, tendon sheath involvement, joint contractures, and proximal muscle weakness.
- Rheumatologic examinations should include searching for tendon friction rubs (TFRs), especially in patients with recent-onset Raynaud phenomenon and swollen fingers, as their presence is important in terms of disease classification, severity, progression, and prognostication.

Continued

Disclosures: Dr Morrisroe is supported by a Royal Australasian College of Physicians Shields Research Entry Scholarship and the Australian Scleroderma Interest Group Fellowship. Dr Nikpour is a recipient of a David Bickart Clinician Research Fellowship from the University of Melbourne Faculty of Medicine, Dentistry and Health Sciences and holds an NHMRC Clinical Early Career Research Fellowship (APP1071735).

[a] Department of Rheumatology, St Vincent's Hospital, 41 Victoria Parade, Level 3 Daly Wing, Fitzroy, Victoria 3065, Australia; [b] Department of Rheumatology, St Vincent's Hospital, 41 Victoria Parade, Fitzroy, Victoria 3065, Australia; [c] Department of Medicine, The University of Melbourne, 41 Victoria Parade, Fitzroy, Victoria 3065, Australia; [d] Rheumatology Unit, Royal Adelaide Hospital, North Terrace, Adelaide 5000, Australia; [e] Discipline of Medicine, University of Adelaide, Adelaide 5000, Australia
* Corresponding author. Department of Rheumatology, St Vincent's Hospital, 41 Victoria Parade, Fitzroy, Victoria 3065, Australia.
E-mail address: m.nikpour@unimelb.edu.au

Continued

- Autoantibodies in SSc frequently characterize distinct phenotypic subsets of disease. Anticyclic citrullinated peptide antibody (ACPA) can predict patients SSc who will develop arthritis and identify patients with scleroderma-rheumatoid arthritis (SSc-RA) overlap syndrome. Anti-polymyositis scleroderma (PM-Scl) antibody is often indicative of an overlap syndrome with an inflammatory myositis and is associated with a more favorable disease course.
- Large controlled randomized trials with adequate follow-up are required to establish treatment guidelines for patients with SSc.

ARTICULAR INVOLVEMENT IN SYSTEMIC SCLEROSIS
Definition

Articular and tendon involvement in SSc is defined by the occurrence of synovitis, arthralgia, and joint contractures, often accompanied by TFRs.[1–12] These manifestations are more likely to occur together in the same patient and are associated with the diffuse cutaneous disease subtype and a more severe disease phenotype.

Prevalence

Articular involvement is common is SSc, eventually affecting 46% to 95% of patients.[13] Data from the European League Against Rheumatism Scleroderma Trial and Research Group (European Scleroderma and Trials and Research group) database indicate point prevalences of 16% for synovitis, 11% for TFRs, and 31% for joint contractures.[14] Hands (particularly the metacarpophalangeal [MCP] and proximal interphalangeal [PIP] joints) and wrists are the most commonly affected joints. Impaired hand function with reduced hand grip due to pain, arthritis, and joint contractures has a significant psychosocial and economic impact on patients by reducing the ability to perform activities of daily living and to participate in work.[11,14] Articular involvement, disability, pain, and unemployment are all independent risk factors for depression in patients with SSc, which occurs with a prevalence of 36% to 65%[15] and is associated with social isolation, worse perception of quality of life, and decreased adherence to medications.

Clinical Features

Generalized arthralgias and stiffness are the most common presentations of joint involvement.[13,14] Clinically evident arthritis occurs in 12% to 65% of patients with SSc. It may be the first manifestations of SSc, preceding even the onset of Raynaud phenomenon, and can cause diagnostic confusion. Hence, it is important to examine for clinical signs of early SSc, such as puffy fingers and nail fold capillary changes in anyone presenting with inflammatory arthritis.

The onset of joint involvement in SSc may be acute or insidious, with an intermittent or chronic course. The pattern of distribution is most commonly polyarticular but can be oligoarticular or monoarticular.[13,14] Effusions, if present, are usually small and occur predominantly in the knee joint.[14] With disease progression, joint contractures due to joint destruction, ankylosis, and dermal fibrotic changes occur in 31% of patients resulting in functional disability. Joint contractures are most apparent at the MCP and interphalangeal joints.[14]

Recent EUSTAR registry data indicate that the frequency of synovitis is significantly higher in patients with diffuse cutaneous disease and that synovitis occurring within 5 years of the first non-Raynaud symptom is predictive of the diffuse disease subset.[14] The presence of synovitis was associated with severe vascular (pulmonary hypertension defined as systolic pulmonary arterial pressure on echocardiogram >40 mm Hg) and muscular (defined as muscle weakness) involvement. Synovitis was also associated with elevated acute phase reactants, indicating more severe systemic inflammation and disease course. Similarly, the prevalence of joint contractures was higher in the diffuse subset and was associated with severe vascular, muscular, and pulmonary interstitial involvement.[14]

Investigations

Laboratory findings

Although rheumatoid factor is present in 30% of patients with SSc, this is nonspecific and does not predict MSK involvement. ACPAs on the other hand, are helpful in identifying those patients with SSc who will develop arthralgia and inflammatory arthritis.[16] In particular, ACPA has a sensitivity of 50% to 100% and specificity of 95% in identifying patients with SSc-RA overlap syndrome.[16,17] SSc-RA overlap is a distinct genetic, clinical, and serologic entity and is uncommon in SSc, with a prevalence of 1% to 5%.[17] However, these patients are more likely to develop bone erosions and joint deformities.

Synovial fluid from SSc arthritis reveals normal or modestly increased leukocyte concentrations (<2000 cells/mm^3) with a predominantly mononuclear infiltrate.[13] Synovial biopsies show evidence of inflammation, with lymphocytic and plasma cell infiltration, associated with focal microvascular obliteration and superficial fibrin deposits. Pannus is rarely present.[13,14] The lack of synovial proliferation and pannus formation in SSc suggests a benign synovitis in comparison with RA.

Imaging

Radiographic findings vary widely in SSc. Distinctive abnormalities include juxtaarticular osteopenia, joint space narrowing, and erosions. A distinct pattern of distribution of erosions occurs in SSc, primarily affecting the MCP joints and the distal interphalangeal joints.[18] Erosions also occur in the wrist, PIP joints, and the first carpometacarpal joint. Erosions are small, discrete, and less invasive than those of RA. Erosions on baseline imaging predict further progression of erosive changes. No independent predictor of erosion progression has yet been identified.

Power Doppler ultrasonography is a useful tool for detecting inflammation, synovial proliferation, synovitis, erosions, calcinosis, and subclinical TFRs in SSc. Ultrasonography preformed on 52 consecutive patients with SSc identified more patients with synovitis and tenosynovitis than clinical examination alone.[19] Given the aforementioned predictive value for the presence of synovitis, ultrasound imaging may have a role in detecting patients at a higher risk of a severe progressive disease phenotype.

MRI demonstrates a high prevalence of inflammatory findings in SSc.[18] In one study, MRI detected synovitis in 47%, tenosynovitis in 47%, erosions in 41%, and bone edema in 53% of patients. None of these inflammatory findings correlated consistently with clinical findings.[20]

Given the burden of MSK manifestations in SSc, their associated morbidity, and lack of evidence-based therapeutic options, randomized trials are required to determine effective treatment regimes. Ultrasonography and MRI could be integrated into these trials to enable adequate patient selection and response to therapy.

TENDON INVOLVEMENT IN SYSTEMIC SCLEROSIS

Tendon abnormalities are a common finding in SSc, including inflammatory proliferative tenosynovitis, tendon rupture, and TFRs. TFRs are defined by a leathery, rubbing, squeaking sensation detected as the tendon is moved actively or passively through its range of action.[13] TFRs occur at a prevalence of 20% in patients with established diffuse disease and in 36% of early diffuse disease. The etiology is unknown but is thought to be secondary to fibrin deposition within tendon synovial sheaths and overlying fascia.[13,21] Pathologic examination demonstrates thickening and fibrinous deposits on the surface of the affected sheaths with little inflammatory reaction. Over time, fibrous deposits develop, leading to audible tendon rubs and flexion contractures.

TFRs occur throughout the body. In the legs, TFRs can be detected over the tendons of tibialis anterior and peroneus muscles and the Achilles tendon. In the forearm, the rub is usually felt over the flexor and extensor muscles proximal to the wrist. Median nerve compression leading to carpal tunnel syndrome can also occur as a consequence of tendon involvement beneath the transverse carpal ligament.[13]

The presence of palpable TFRs is associated with active disease and is a significant predictor of severe diffuse cutaneous involvement; internal organ involvement, including renal, muscular, and cardiac manifestations; and increased mortality.[1,13,21] The presence of TFRs is independently associated with digital ulceration, muscle weakness, pulmonary fibrosis, proteinuria, and active disease.[14,22] The occurrence of TFRs in early disease is associated with more severe disease regardless of the disease subtype.[14] Therefore, searching for TFRs should be part of every rheumatologic examination, especially in patients with recent onset of Raynaud phenomenon and swollen fingers, as the presence of TFRs is important in terms of disease classification, severity, progression, and prognostication.

Clinical examination often underestimates the presence of tenosynovitis, which can be further characterized by ultrasonography or MRI, although the place of these modalities in the assessment of tendon involvement in SSc is yet to be defined.

CALCINOSIS IN SYSTEMIC SCLEROSIS

Involvement of digits by the vascular abnormalities and fibrosis that characterize SSc results in digital ischemia and sclerodactyly, often with contractures and ulceration over the extensor aspects of the interphalangeal joints (**Figs. 1–4**). It is a major contributor to morbidity, disability, and pain. In addition, a significant proportion of patients develop subcutaneous calcinosis, which can ulcerate through the skin, causing pain, disability, and infection (see **Figs. 2** and **3**).

Calcinosis is the deposition of amorphous calcium hydroxyapatite crystals in subcutaneous tissues and occurs in both limited and diffuse disease with a prevalence of 25%.[23] Deposits are most commonly found in the hands but can occur anywhere including wrists, forearms, elbows, shoulders, around the iliac crests and gluteal region, and along the spine.[23] When calcinosis occurs on the distal phalanx, digital ulceration and secondary infection can occur. Calcinosis is seen radiographically as multilocular masses of calcium density that can display fluid levels of different densities (see **Figs. 1** and **2**).

If calcinosis causes severe pain, recurrent infection or ulceration, functional joint impairment, or nerve compression, surgical excision could be considered. Even after surgery, recurrences are common. There are no clear recommendations for pharmacotherapy.[24]

BONE INVOLVEMENT IN SYSTEMIC SCLEROSIS

Bone involvement in SSc is characterized by resorption of the terminal tuft of the phalanx (acro-osteolysis), occurring in 20% to 25% of patients, more frequently in the hands than in the feet.[25] This condition is often accompanied by acral soft-tissue

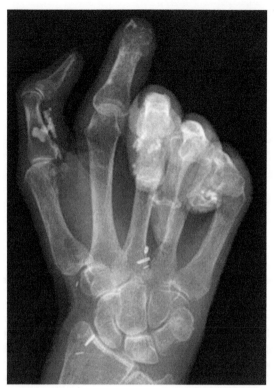

Fig. 1. Hand radiograph in patient with systemic sclerosis showing calcinosis, acro-osteolysis, and joint contractures.

thinning or pulp atrophy. Bone resorption begins at the tuft, particularly on the palmer surface of the bone and progressively leads to sharpening of the phalanx (see **Fig. 1**). At times, a pencil in cup deformity similar to that of psoriatic arthritis occurs, suggesting that SSc erosions have an entheseal origin.[1] In severe cases, reduction in finger length results from destruction of all of the distal phalanges. Rarely proximal phalanx bone resorption occurs.

The exact etiology of acro-osteolysis is unknown. It is thought that the combination of digital ischemia from impaired blood supply and retractile pressure from skin

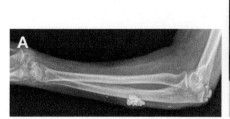
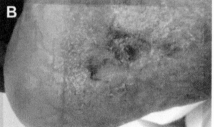

Fig. 2. (*A*) Radiograph of forearm of patient with systemic sclerosis showing calcinosis. (*B*) Elbow of the same patient showing ulceration overlying the area of calcinosis.

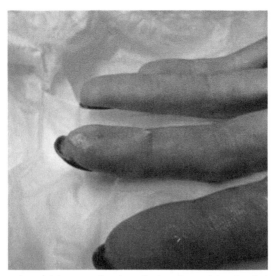

Fig. 3. Hand of a patient with systemic sclerosis showing calcinosis of the fingers.

thickening leads to ischemic atrophy resulting in distal tuft resorption.[1] Patients with severe digital ischemia develop fingertip ulcers and digital pitting, and it seems reasonable to propose that soft-tissue loss is paralleled by bone loss. This theory is further strengthened by a study showing that moderate-severe acro-osteolysis was significantly associated with severe digital ischemia with a graded response.[25] Moderate-severe acro-osteolysis was also associated with a longer duration of Raynaud phenomenon and severe calcinosis on radiography. Acro-osteolysis has previously been reported to be associated with both digital calcinosis and secondary hyperparathyroidism.[26]

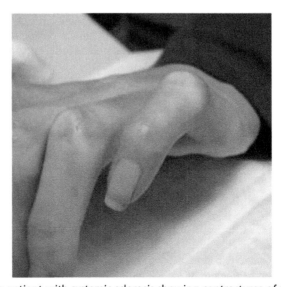

Fig. 4. Hand of a patient with systemic sclerosis showing contractures of the fingers.

Radiographic manifestations of bone involvement in the hands and their corresponding frequency include erosions (21%), joint space narrowing (28%), concomitant erosions and joint space narrowing (18%), radiologic demineralization (23%), acro-osteolysis (22%), flexion contractures (27%), and calcinosis (23%).[1]

Imaging modalities for assessment of bone involvement include radiography and MRI. Radiographic changes include demineralization, which is associated with arthritis and systemic inflammation, hyperostosis of the phalangeal tuft, and the resorption of bone at various sites, including the carpal bones, distal radius and ulna, clavicles, ribs, and spine.[18] MRI depicts bone resorption whereby resorbed bone is replaced by fibrous tissue.

Low bone density is not an infrequent finding in SSc. Numerous studies to determine whether patients with SSc have an increased risk of osteopenia and/or osteoporosis have reported conflicting results. In addition, many patients with SSc have several concomitant traditional risk factors for low bone density, including increased age, female gender, postmenopausal state, and the use of corticosteroids. Increased fracture risk has been identified in other rheumatic conditions such as RA, but this is yet to be confirmed in SSc.[27]

MYOPATHY IN SYSTEMIC SCLEROSIS
Definition

SSc myopathy is a heterogeneous group of muscle disorders occurring among patients with SSc. It encompasses several biological processes that occur at the intersection of rheumatologic and neuromuscular disorders, including weakness secondary to inflammatory myositis (indistinguishable from polymyositis) or a noninflammatory myopathy.[12]

No uniform classification criteria exist for SSc myopathy. The most commonly used diagnostic criteria include muscle weakness, myalgia, and elevation of creatine kinase (CK) levels more than 5 times the upper limit of normal, together with electromyographic (EMG) or histologic evidence of muscle involvement.[28]

Prevalence

Because of the disparate diagnostic criteria, the prevalence of SSc myopathy has varied widely between studies, ranging from 14% to 96%.[1,12] SSc myositis has a more clearly defined prevalence of 10% to 15%.[12,29]

Clinical Features

In 2009, a multicenter French study evaluated 35 patients (30 women, 5 men) with SSc to elucidate the clinical and pathologic features of scleroderma myopathy.[28] The median time from diagnosis of SSc to onset of myopathy was 5 years (range 0–23 years), and most patients (75%) had diffuse SSc. The most common clinical manifestations included symmetric proximal muscle weakness (77%), myalgia (86%), and elevated levels of CK (82%) and aldolase (76%).

Investigations

If scleroderma myopathy is suspected, muscle strength should be evaluated clinically with the 8-manual muscle testing scale, which examines proximal and distal muscle strength in the arms, legs, and truncal muscles. Measurements can be monitored over time for improvement, stability, or deterioration.

Serologic markers include CK, aldolase, and lactate dehydrogenase.[12] Aldolase has been suggested as a novel biomarker for predicting asymptomatic patients with SSc who will develop SSc myopathy.[12,30] In a prospective study, an elevated aldolase level, of all the above-mentioned serologic markers, had the highest predictive power with a sensitivity of 89% and specificity of 67%.[30]

EMG confirms the presence of a myopathic process, which is the most common finding in SSc myopathy occurring in 93% of patients with SSc myositis.[28]

MRI also aids in the detection of myositis. On T2-weighted images, symmetric, bilateral high-intensity signal indicating muscle edema is often seen in the girdle muscles.[1,28] Muscle atrophy and fatty infiltration can be seen in chronic myositis.[1,28] Perifascial enhancement and muscular edema on MRI are the most strongly correlated with muscle weakness.[31]

Muscle biopsy is the diagnostic gold standard. The most frequent histologic finding is mononuclear inflammation at septal or perimysial, endomysial, and/or perivascular areas. Infiltrate is composed of CD4 T cells, B cells, and complement deposits on vascular walls. Over time, this inflammation progresses to fibrosis and necrosis.[28]

Electrocardiography and echocardiography are strongly recommended, as there is a strong correlation between SSc myopathy and myocardial disease.[1,32]

Prognosis

SSc myopathy is associated with cardiopulmonary complications leading to increased mortality.[28] Pulmonary complications, including interstitial lung disease and pulmonary hypertension, are the leading cause of death for patients with SSc myopathy.[32]

After 4.5 years of follow-up, 24% to 69% of patients in the French study had a complete or partial muscle remission.[28] Histologic muscle inflammation was associated with good muscle prognosis in multivariable analysis (odds ratio [OR], ~45; 95% confidence interval [CI], 3–705) in addition to histologic evidence of necrosis (OR, 16.5; 95% CI, 1.3–208). Patients without muscle inflammation had a poorer outcome after corticosteroid treatment (38% favorable response vs 90% in patients with inflammation).

In a study published by the Canadian Scleroderma Research Group, patients with SSc with an elevated CK level were more likely to be male and younger and to have diffuse disease, TFRs, a forced vital capacity less than 70%, positive ribonucleoprotein antibody and topoisomerase 1 antibody, higher skin score, higher Health Assessment Questionnaire (HAQ) scores, and worse survival at 1, 3, and 10 years. The most common causes of death were interstitial lung disease, pulmonary arterial hypertension, and cardiac involvement.[32]

Anti-polymyositis Scleroderma Antibody in Systemic Sclerosis Myopathy

Autoantibodies in SSc frequently characterize distinct phenotypic subsets of disease. Anti-PM-Scl antibody positivity often indicates an overlap syndrome most commonly with an inflammatory myositis. The prevalence of this antibody in SSc is 5% to 7.5%, with greater than 50% having no other SSc-specific antibody.

Koschik and colleagues[33] examined the disease manifestations and mortality risk among those with and without anti-PM-Scl antibody. Seropositivity conferred different disease manifestations and improved survival compared with seronegative patients. Patients with anti-PM-Scl antibody were younger at SSc symptom onset (38 ± 18 vs 43 ± 15 years); had more limited skin disease (72% vs 52%, P = .001); were more likely to have skeletal muscle involvement (51% vs 14%, P<.0001), subcutaneous calcinosis (P<.003), and pulmonary fibrosis (50% vs 37%, P = .04); and were less likely to have gastrointestinal involvement (52% vs 79%, P = .0001). Seropositivity conferred an overall survival benefit, with a 10-year cumulative survival rate of 91% versus 65%, respectively; P = .0002. After adjusting for age, sex, and disease subtype, patients with anti-PM-Scl had a reduced risk of death (hazard ratio [HR], 0.3; 95% CI, 0.1–0.7, P = .0006). These results are consistent with other reports.[12,34,35]

THERAPY FOR MUSCULOSKELETAL MANIFESTATIONS OF SYSTEMIC SCLEROSIS

There are no randomized controlled trials evaluating therapies for relief of symptoms or disease-modifying agents in the treatment of SSc MSK manifestations. Furthermore, there are no agreed and validated outcome measures for measuring MSK manifestations of SSc, with the exception of the HAQ disability index (HAQ-DI). Indirect measures of the impact of MSK disease include the scleroderma HAQ-DI and short form 36 health survey.

Pharmacologic management to date has been supportive and symptomatic.[13] Arthralgias can be treated with judicious use of nonsteroidal anti-inflammatory agents in patients without severe gastroesophageal reflux disease, gastric antral vascular ectasia, and renal or cardiac dysfunction. Inflammatory arthritis can be treated with low-dose corticosteroids (<10 mg/d); however, caution must be exercised in those patients at risk of renal crisis.[36] The use of methotrexate in SSc arthritis is based on evidence of benefit in RA. In SSc, subcutaneous or intramuscular administration may be more efficacious given the potential for malabsorption.[37]

Intravenous immunoglobulin (IVIG) therapy may have a role in severe refractory inflammatory arthritis, as it reduced joint pain and tenderness and improved quality of life in a small 6-month pilot study of 7 women.[38]

Biological disease modifying antirheumatic drugs (DMARDs), such as tumor necrosis factor (TNF) inhibitors, are effective for inflammatory joint disease such as RA. There is a paucity of data regarding their efficacy and safety in the treatment of MSK manifestations in SSc, but a small retrospective review of 10 patients with SSc and refractory arthritis treated with a TNF inhibitor for more than 12 months showed a significant reduction in the median swollen and tender joint counts at 3 months and reduction in pain scores.[39] These findings have been replicated in other studies.[40,41] Of concern, 30% of patients developed a malignancy,[39] a finding that requires further investigation. Tocilizumab, an interleukin 6 receptor blocker, and abatacept, a costimulatory signal modulator, were found to be safe and efficacious in treating refractory SSc arthritis in a small observational study of 20 patients.[42]

Rituximab, a chimeric monoclonal antibody to CD20 on B cells, is efficacious in RA,[43] but no study has been performed to evaluate its use in the MSK manifestations of SSc.

Large controlled randomized trials with adequate follow-up to determine the efficacy and safety of biological DMARDs are needed to enable the establishment of treatment guidelines.

Options for nonpharmacologic management to improve joint motion, hand function, and cardiopulmonary endurance include physiotherapy and rehabilitation techniques, such as paraffin wax treatment, hand and face stretching exercises, connective tissue massage and joint manipulation, aerobic exercise, and resistance training.[13]

Hand surgery is an option for pain relief, with repositioning of the digits and fusion in a functional position providing a modest gain in mobility.[44] Postoperative wound healing is a particular concern. If surgery is contemplated, referral to a hand surgeon with experience in SSc is advisable and local or regional anesthesia is recommended for patients with clinically significant cardiac and/or pulmonary comorbidities.

The treatment of SSc myopathy is similar to that of other inflammatory myopathies. SSc myositis is thought to initially be caused by inflammation, which untreated progresses to fibrosis and muscle atrophy. The initial treatment regimen includes both corticosteroids and DMARDs, such as methotrexate and azathioprine. Once inflammation is controlled, nonpharmacologic therapy such as physiotherapy and rehabilitation techniques can be instituted to increase muscle strength. Partial or complete responses in refractory myositis have been reported with IVIG and biological DMARDs, including abatacept and rituximab, in case series.[42,45-47]

SUMMARY

MSK involvement in scleroderma is common and is associated with significant disability and psychosocial and economic burden. These manifestations pose particular challenges for the treating clinician given the paucity of data to help guide effective treatment. Synovitis and TFRs may be the first indication of early diffuse SSc and may aid in identifying patients with a higher risk disease phenotype. The goals of future work in this area should include developing a validated outcome measure for MSK manifestations of SSc to enable large clinical trials to assess the efficacy of existing drugs in SSc and to identify new drugs, allowing a reduction in disease morbidity and improvement in quality of life.

ACKNOWLEDGMENTS

The authors thank Dr Wendy Stevens and Barbara Gemmell for contributing some of the images included in this article.

REFERENCES

1. Randone SB, Guiducci S, Cerinic MM. Musculoskeletal involvement in systemic sclerosis. Best Pract Res Clin Rheumatol 2008;22(2):339–50.
2. Casas JA, Subauste CP, Alarcon GS. A new promising treatment in systemic sclerosis: 5-fluorouracil. Ann Rheum Dis 1987;46(10):763–7.
3. Furst DE, Clements PJ, Hillis S, et al. Immunosuppression with chlorambucil, versus placebo, for scleroderma. Results of a three-year, parallel, randomized, double-blind study. Arthritis Rheum 1989;32(5):584–93.
4. Geirsson AJ, Wollheim FA, Akesson A. Disease severity of 100 patients with systemic sclerosis over a period of 14 years: using a modified Medsger scale. Ann Rheum Dis 2001;60(12):1117–22.
5. Hughes P, Holt S, Rowell NR, et al. Thymus-dependent (T) lymphocyte deficiency in progressive systemic sclerosis. Br J Dermatol 1976;95(5):469–73.
6. Medsger TA Jr, Bombardieri S, Czirjak L, et al. Assessment of disease severity and prognosis. Clin Exp Rheumatol 2003;21(3 Suppl 29):S42–6.
7. Medsger TA Jr, Silman AJ, Steen VD, et al. A disease severity scale for systemic sclerosis: development and testing. J Rheumatol 1999;26(10):2159–67.
8. Minier T, Nagy Z, Balint Z, et al. Construct validity evaluation of the European Scleroderma Study Group activity index, and investigation of possible new disease activity markers in systemic sclerosis. Rheumatology (Oxford) 2010;49(6):1133–45.
9. Morita Y, Muro Y, Sugiura K, et al. Results of the Health Assessment Questionnaire for Japanese patients with systemic sclerosis–measuring functional impairment in systemic sclerosis versus other connective tissue diseases. Clin Exp Rheumatol 2007;25(3):367–72.
10. Valentini G, Della Rossa A, Bombardieri S, et al. European multicentre study to define disease activity criteria for systemic sclerosis. II. Identification of disease activity variables and development of preliminary activity indexes. Ann Rheum Dis 2001;60(6):592–8.

11. Bassel M, Hudson M, Taillefer SS, et al. Frequency and impact of symptoms experienced by patients with systemic sclerosis: results from a Canadian National Survey. Rheumatology (Oxford) 2011;50(4):762–7.

12. Paik JJ, Mammen AL, Wigley FM, et al. Myopathy in scleroderma, its identification, prevalence, and treatment: lessons learned from cohort studies. Curr Opin Rheumatol 2014;26(2):124–30.

13. Avouac J, Clements PJ, Khanna D, et al. Articular involvement in systemic sclerosis. Rheumatology (Oxford) 2012;51(8):1347–56.

14. Avouac J, Walker U, Tyndall A, et al. Characteristics of joint involvement and relationships with systemic inflammation in systemic sclerosis: results from the EULAR Scleroderma Trial and Research Group (EUSTAR) database. J Rheumatol 2010;37(7):1488–501.

15. Tedeschini E, Pingani L, Simoni E, et al. Correlation of articular involvement, skin disfigurement and unemployment with depressive symptoms in patients with systemic sclerosis: a hospital sample. Int J Rheum Dis 2014;17(2):186–94.

16. Polimeni M, Feniman D, Skare TS, et al. Anti-cyclic citrullinated peptide antibodies in scleroderma patients. Clin Rheumatol 2012;31(5):877–80.

17. Ueda-Hayakawa I, Hasegawa M, Kumada S, et al. Usefulness of anti-cyclic citrullinated peptide antibody and rheumatoid factor to detect rheumatoid arthritis in patients with systemic sclerosis. Rheumatology (Oxford) 2010;49(11):2135–9.

18. Chapin R, Hant FN. Imaging of scleroderma. Rheum Dis Clin North Am 2013; 39(3):515–46.

19. Elhai M, Guerini H, Bazeli R, et al. Ultrasonographic hand features in systemic sclerosis and correlates with clinical, biologic, and radiographic findings. Arthritis Care Res 2012;64(8):1244–9.

20. Low AH, Lax M, Johnson SR, et al. Magnetic resonance imaging of the hand in systemic sclerosis. J Rheumatol 2009;36(5):961–4.

21. Stoenoiu MS, Houssiau FA, Lecouvet FE. Tendon friction rubs in systemic sclerosis: a possible explanation–an ultrasound and magnetic resonance imaging study. Rheumatology (Oxford) 2013;52(3):529–33.

22. Khanna PP, Furst DE, Clements PJ, et al. Tendon friction rubs in early diffuse systemic sclerosis: prevalence, characteristics and longitudinal changes in a randomized controlled trial. Rheumatology (Oxford) 2010;49(5):955–9.

23. Daumas A, Rossi P, Ariey-Bonnet D, et al. Generalized calcinosis in systemic sclerosis. QJM 2014;107(3):219–21.

24. Cukierman T, Elinav E, Korem M, et al. Low dose warfarin treatment for calcinosis in patients with systemic sclerosis. Ann Rheum Dis 2004;63(10):1341–3.

25. Johnstone EM, Hutchinson CE, Vail A, et al. Acro-osteolysis in systemic sclerosis is associated with digital ischaemia and severe calcinosis. Rheumatology (Oxford) 2012;51(12):2234–8.

26. Braun-Moscovici Y, Furst DE, Markovits D, et al. Vitamin D, parathyroid hormone, and acro-osteolysis in systemic sclerosis. J Rheumatol 2008;35(11):2201–5.

27. Omair MA, Pagnoux C, McDonald-Blumer H, et al. Low bone density in systemic sclerosis. A systematic review. J Rheumatol 2013;40(11):1881–90.

28. Ranque B, Authier FJ, Le-Guern V, et al. A descriptive and prognostic study of systemic sclerosis-associated myopathies. Ann Rheum Dis 2009;68(9):1474–7.

29. Muangchan C, Baron M, Pope J. The 15% rule in scleroderma: the frequency of severe organ complications in systemic sclerosis. A systematic review. J Rheumatol 2013;40(9):1545–56.

30. Toledano C, Gain M, Kettaneh A, et al. Aldolase predicts subsequent myopathy occurrence in systemic sclerosis. Arthritis Res Ther 2012;14(3):R152.

31. Schanz S, Henes J, Ulmer A, et al. Magnetic resonance imaging findings in patients with systemic scleroderma and musculoskeletal symptoms. Eur Radiol 2013;23(1):212–21.

32. Jung M, Bonner A, Hudson M, et al. Myopathy is a poor prognostic feature in systemic sclerosis: results from the Canadian Scleroderma Research Group (CSRG) cohort. Scand J Rheumatol 2014;43(3):217–20.

33. Koschik RW 2nd, Fertig N, Lucas MR, et al. Anti-PM-Scl antibody in patients with systemic sclerosis. Clin Exp Rheumatol 2012;30(2 Suppl 71):S12–6.

34. Vandergheynst F, Ocmant A, Sordet C, et al. Anti-PM/Scl antibodies in connective tissue disease: clinical and biological assessment of 14 patients. Clin Exp Rheumatol 2006;24(2):129–33.

35. D'Aoust J, Hudson M, Tatibouet S, et al. Clinical and serologic correlates of anti-PM/Scl antibodies in systemic sclerosis: a multicenter study of 763 patients. Arthritis Rheumatol 2014;66(6):1608–15.

36. Steen VD, Medsger TA Jr. Case-control study of corticosteroids and other drugs that either precipitate or protect from the development of scleroderma renal crisis. Arthritis Rheum 1998;41(9):1613–9.

37. Visser K, van der Heijde D. Optimal dosage and route of administration of methotrexate in rheumatoid arthritis: a systematic review of the literature. Ann Rheum Dis 2009;68(7):1094–9.

38. Nacci F, Righi A, Conforti ML, et al. Intravenous immunoglobulins improve the function and ameliorate joint involvement in systemic sclerosis: a pilot study. Ann Rheum Dis 2007;66(7):977–9.

39. Omair MA, Phumethum V, Johnson SR. Long-term safety and effectiveness of tumour necrosis factor inhibitors in systemic sclerosis patients with inflammatory arthritis. Clin Exp Rheumatol 2012;30(2 Suppl 71):S55–9.

40. Phumethum V, Jamal S, Johnson SR. Biologic therapy for systemic sclerosis: a systematic review. J Rheumatol 2011;38(2):289–96.

41. Lam GK, Hummers LK, Woods A, et al. Efficacy and safety of etanercept in the treatment of scleroderma-associated joint disease. J Rheumatol 2007;34(7): 1636–7.

42. Elhai M, Meunier M, Matucci-Cerinic M, et al. Outcomes of patients with systemic sclerosis-associated polyarthritis and myopathy treated with tocilizumab or abatacept: a EUSTAR observational study. Ann Rheum Dis 2013;72(7):1217–20.

43. Hernandez-Cruz B, Garcia-Arias M, Ariza Ariza R, et al. Rituximab in rheumatoid arthritis: a systematic review of efficacy and safety. Reumatol Clin 2011;7(5): 314–22 [in Spanish].

44. Anandacoomarasamy A, Englert H, Manolios N, et al. Reconstructive hand surgery for scleroderma joint contractures. J Hand Surg 2007;32(7):1107–12.

45. Wang DX, Shu XM, Tian XL, et al. Intravenous immunoglobulin therapy in adult patients with polymyositis/dermatomyositis: a systematic literature review. Clin Rheumatol 2012;31(5):801–6.

46. Fabri M, Hunzelmann N, Krieg T, et al. Discordant response to rituximab in a systemic sclerosis patient with associated myositis. J Am Acad Dermatol 2008;58(5 Suppl 1):S127–8.

47. Arkfeld DG. The potential utility of B cell-directed biologic therapy in autoimmune diseases. Rheumatol Int 2008;28(3):205–15.

Psychosocial Aspects of Scleroderma

Linda Kwakkenbos, PhD[a,b,*], Vanessa C. Delisle, MSc[a,c], Rina S. Fox, MS, MPH[d], Shadi Gholizadeh, MSc[d], Lisa R. Jewett, MSc[a,c], Brooke Levis, MSc[a,e], Katherine Milette, MA[a,c], Sarah D. Mills, MS[d], Vanessa L. Malcarne, PhD[d,f], Brett D. Thombs, PhD[a,b,c,e,g,h,i]

KEYWORDS

- Scleroderma • Systemic sclerosis • Psychosocial • Quality of life
- Self-management

KEY POINTS

- Symptoms of systemic sclerosis (SSc), including fatigue, pain, pruritus, sleep problems, and sexual impairments, negatively influence quality of life in many patients, and may lead to emotional consequences such as depression, anxiety, and body image distress caused by appearance changes.
- Providing accessible information to patients with SSc regarding problems common to people living with the disease, as well as information regarding useful resources and services to address these problems, can help patients with SSc and can easily be implemented by health care professionals.

Continued

Conflicts of Interest: The authors have no conflicts of interest to disclose.

Disclosure: This work was supported by a grant from the Canadian Institutes of Health Research (CIHR; #TR3-267681). Dr L. Kwakkenbos was supported by a Fonds de la Recherche en Santé Québec (FRSQ) postdoctoral fellowship. Ms V.C. Delisle, Ms L.R. Jewett, and Ms K. Milette were supported by CIHR Doctoral Research Awards. Ms B. Levis was supported by an FRSQ Doctoral Training Award. Dr B.D. Thombs was supported by an Investigator Salary Award from the Arthritis Society.

[a] Lady Davis Institute for Medical Research, Jewish General Hospital, 4333 Cote Ste Catherine Road, Montréal, Québec H3T 1E4, Canada; [b] Department of Psychiatry, McGill University, 1033 Pine Avenue West, Montréal, Québec H3A 1A1, Canada; [c] Department of Educational and Counselling Psychology, McGill University, 3700 McTavish Street, Montréal, Québec H3A 1Y2, Canada; [d] San Diego Joint Doctoral Program in Clinical Psychology, San Diego State University, University of California, 6363 Alvarado Court, San Diego, CA 92120-4913, USA; [e] Department of Epidemiology, Biostatistics, and Occupational Health, McGill University, 1020 Pine Avenue West, Montréal, Québec H3A 1A2, Canada; [f] Department of Psychology, San Diego State University, 5500 Campanile Drive, San Diego, CA 92182-4611, USA; [g] Department of Medicine, McGill University, 3655 Sir William Osler, Montréal, Québec H3G 1Y6, Canada; [h] Department of Psychology, McGill University, 1205 Dr. Penfield Avenue, Montréal, Québec H3A 1B1, Canada; [i] School of Nursing, McGill University, 3506 University Street, Montréal, Québec H3A 2A7, Canada

* Corresponding author. Jewish General Hospital, 4333 Cote Sainte Catherine Road, Montreal, Quebec H3T 1E4, Canada.

E-mail address: kwakkenbosl@gmail.com

Continued

- In addition to referrals for professional health care interventions, low-intensity strategies such as self-management programs and support groups may be helpful to some patients with SSc.
- Future research should focus on the development and testing of interventions designed specifically to meet the educational and psychosocial needs of patients with SSc.

INTRODUCTION

Systemic sclerosis (SSc; also called scleroderma) has far-reaching consequences for physical health, as well as emotional and social well-being.[1–4] Because there is no known cure for the disease, SSc treatment focuses on reducing symptoms and disability, and improving health-related quality of life (HRQL). This article summarizes the impact of SSc on common patient-reported problems associated with HRQL and describes potential interventions to support coping with the consequences of the disease.

Depression

Depression involves symptoms that may include sadness, loss of interest or pleasure, feelings of guilt or low self-esteem, poor concentration, and disturbed sleep or appetite. A study of 345 patients with SSc enrolled in a Canadian registry reported that the prevalence of major depressive disorder (MDD) was 4% for the past 30 days, 11% for the past 12 months, and 23% for lifetime.[5] A French study of 50 hospitalized patients with SSc and 50 patients with SSc who attended a patient organization meeting found that 19% had current MDD and 56% had lifetime MDD, and rates were higher in hospitalized (28% current) versus nonhospitalized (10% current) patients.[6] Depression is substantially more common in patients with SSc than in the general population and may be more prevalent than in other rheumatic diseases.[5] However, many patients with SSc and other chronic diseases who meet criteria for MDD at a given time point do not meet criteria consistently. In the Canadian sample, only 3 of 12 patients with SSc who had a current major depressive episode at baseline met diagnostic criteria 1 month later.[7] Some episodes may be time limited and may resolve without targeted intervention or treatment. Others may reflect ongoing moderate symptoms that only variably meet criteria for formal diagnosis. Many patients with SSc describe ongoing emotional distress from the burden of living with the disease, but differentiate this qualitatively from what they consider clinical depression.[8] Cross sectionally, factors associated with symptoms of depression in SSc include greater overall disease burden, which may involve degree of gastrointestinal involvement; breathing problems; skin involvement; and tender joints.[9–11]

Anxiety and Fear

Anxiety can be a normal reaction to stress; however, it may also lead to mental health problems when experienced in excess. To date, only 1 study documented the prevalence of anxiety disorders among patients with SSc. In that study, 49% of 50 hospitalized patients and 50 patients who attended a patient meeting had at least 1 current anxiety disorder, and 64% met criteria for at least 1 anxiety disorder in their lifetimes. Social anxiety and generalized anxiety disorder were the most common.[6] There was no difference in prevalence between hospitalized and nonhospitalized patients.

The course of SSc is highly unpredictable and patients may perceive the future as uncertain. For patients, worry about the future, including fear of disease progression, fear of becoming physically disabled, and fear of being dependent on others, is an important source of stress.[12,13] Because SSc is unpredictable and associated with serious consequences, these concerns are realistic and in themselves do not represent anxiety disorders, for which irrational fear is typically a central component.[13] Nonetheless, fear of progression can affect HRQL substantially. In a cross-sectional study of 215 patients with SSc from the Netherlands, fear of progression was highly associated with symptoms of depression.[13]

Fatigue

Fatigue from a chronic medical disease is characterized by persistent exhaustion that is disproportionate to exertion and not relieved by rest.[14] Fatigue is the most commonly experienced symptom of SSc and has a substantial impact on HRQL, as well as the ability to perform daily activities, including work.[1,4,15–17] In one Canadian study, 89% of 464 patients with SSc reported fatigue at least some of the time, and 81% of these patients indicated that fatigue had at least a moderate impact on their daily function.[15] Levels of fatigue in SSc are similar to those experienced by patients with other rheumatic diseases and by patients with cancer undergoing active treatment.[18] Cross sectionally, greater fatigue in SSc is associated with increased medical comorbidities, current smoking, pain, breathing problems, and gastrointestinal symptoms.[14] Longitudinally, fatigue severity has been associated with pain; severity of gastrointestinal involvement; and psychological variables, specifically ineffective coping skills.[19]

Sleep

Significant sleep disruption is common in SSc and has broad implications for patients.[15,20–22] A polysomnography study of 27 patients with SSc found that, compared with age-adjusted norms, patients with SSc had reduced sleep efficiency and rapid eye movement sleep, as well as increased arousal and slow wave sleep.[20] Sleep disruption was associated with esophageal dyskinesia and dyspnea, which are common complications of SSc, as well as restless legs syndrome.[20] Observational studies have linked dyspnea, pain, fatigue, pruritus, gastrointestinal symptoms, and depressive symptoms with self-reported poor sleep quality and sleep disruption in SSc.[21,22]

Pain

Between 60% and 83% of patients with SSc report experiencing pain at any given time, and pain levels in SSc are similar to levels reported in chronic pain and rheumatic conditions.[15,23,24] Pain in SSc is associated with reduced HRQL, functional disability, work disability, sleep problems, and symptoms of depression.[22–25] Patients with SSc describe their pain as both localized and generalized in quality,[26] and sources can include pain from Raynaud phenomenon, gastrointestinal pain, joint and musculoskeletal pain, skin pain, and pain caused by calcinosis and ulcers.[1,23,26] Pain ratings are higher among patients with diffuse SSc compared with patients with limited disease, although this difference is generally small.[23] Based on patient reports, overall pain levels are associated with sleep problems, fatigue, and symptoms of depression, as well as physical function, reduced ability to perform daily activities, work disability, and poorer HRQL.[22,23,25,27] How patients with SSc describe their pain and the degree to which they think they can manage it often reflects psychosocial factors, which should be considered in assessment and intervention, especially as related to pharmacologic treatment.[28]

Pruritus

Pruritus, or itch, is common in SSc and is associated with HRQL, even after controlling for sociodemographic and other SSc symptom variables.[29,30] Overall, 43% of 959 patients with SSc from a Canadian registry reported pruritus on most days in the last month.[31] This rate was slightly higher, but not statistically significant, among patients with early SSc (<5 years since onset of non-Raynaud symptoms, 46%) versus those with longer disease duration (≥5 years, 41%).[31] The presence of pruritus is more common among patients with greater skin and gastrointestinal involvement.[31]

Body Image

Acquired disfigurement from an injury or medical illness is often linked to problems with body image, including social avoidance.[32] Appearance changes in highly visible areas of the body, particularly the face and hands, are common in patients with SSc and contribute to body image distress, which in turn can be associated with symptoms of anxiety and depression.[1,4,32–36] Several cross-sectional studies have reported that appearance changes of the face, including changes to the mouth, as well as hand involvement, including skin thickening, have consistently been related to body image distress, including dissatisfaction with appearance, decreased appearance self-esteem, and symptoms of anxiety and depression.[32–36] Other appearance changes, including telangiectasias, may also be associated with body image distress.[36,37] Social discomfort caused by changes in appearance is also related to age.[36] Younger patients, for whom the importance of meeting new people and developing intimate relationships is more pronounced, may experience a greater negative impact of appearance changes on social relationships.[36]

Sexual Function

Sexual dysfunction is a common problem among women with SSc.[1,38–43] Compared with women in the general population, women with SSc are significantly less likely to be sexually active, and sexually active women with SSc are significantly more likely to be sexually impaired.[39,40,42] Factors that are independently associated with being sexually active include younger age, fewer gastrointestinal symptoms, and less severe Raynaud phenomenon symptoms.[41] Among women who are sexually active, sexual impairment is associated with older age, as well as with more severe skin involvement and breathing problems. Vaginal pain is 8 times as common among women with impairment compared with those without.[41]

Among men with SSc, erectile dysfunction (ED) is common with onset typically occurring several years after the manifestation of the first non-Raynaud symptoms.[44–46] In the general population, ED is typically associated with atherosclerosis, but in SSc penile blood flow is impaired because of both myointimal proliferation of small arteries and corporal fibrosis.[46] Men with SSc who have ED are significantly more likely to be older than those without ED and tend to report non-SSc risk factors (eg, alcohol consumption) at higher rates.[45,46] SSc factors associated with ED include severe cutaneous, muscular, or renal involvement; diffuse disease; increased pulmonary pressures; restrictive lung disease;, endothelial dysfunction; and microvascular damage.[45–47] Most men with SSc who have ED do not receive treatment.[45] Among those who do, sildenafil seems to be commonly used, but its efficacy has not been established in SSc.[44,45]

CLINICAL MANAGEMENT

In addition to the core medical treatment of SSc-related symptoms, providing services and interventions to help manage the psychological, behavioral, and social aspects of living with the disease is an important component of patient-centered care. However, there are challenges related to the development, testing, and delivery of such patient-centered interventions in SSc, including the small number of patients and the limited resources available.[2,3] Nonetheless, these types of psychosocial interventions have proved to be effective in reducing disability and improving HRQL in more common conditions, including rheumatic diseases,[48,49] and can reasonably be implemented in SSc.

Stepped-care models for psychological, behavioral, and educational interventions involve matching interventions of differing intensities to patient needs. In general, stepped care starts with the simplest, least intrusive intervention and proceeds to more intense treatment approaches as deemed necessary.[1] Self-help can be a useful first step toward addressing mild problems associated with psychosocial functioning and HRQL. Providing accessible information to both patients and those who support them regarding issues common to people living with SSc, as well as information regarding useful resources and services to address such problems, can be easily implemented by health care professionals. Health care professionals should be aware of the important concerns that affect HRQL in order to help patients to access appropriate resources and facilitate conversations that address concerns of individual patients. In addition, links to other sources of information can be provided in clinics regarding self-help programs that are available, as a first step in providing psychosocial support.

In the context of stepped care, low-intensity interventions are appropriate for people with less severe psychological concerns. However, referral to professional services is needed for patients with more complex or serious psychological problems, such as severe depression, or when lower intensity methods do not work well. For these patients, a focused evaluation of their psychological symptoms and more intense intervention services provided by a mental health professional are often required.

Low-intensity strategies that have been proved effective to improve coping with the consequences of more common chronic diseases, and that may be readily available to many patients with SSc, include self-management programs and support groups.[48,49]

Self-management

Across more prevalent diseases, supportive care programs, such as self-management programs, are increasingly included as core components of patient-centered care. Although there is currently no gold-standard definition, the term self-management has been defined as the ability of patients to manage the symptoms, treatment, physical consequences, psychological consequences, and lifestyle changes inherent in living with a chronic condition. Effective self-management involves the patients' ability to monitor their own condition and to have the cognitive, behavioral, and emotional responses necessary to maintain a satisfactory HRQL.[50]

In more prevalent diseases, such as arthritis, asthma, and diabetes, self-management interventions have been shown to provide benefits to participants in terms of knowledge, performance of self-management behaviors, self-efficacy, and health status.[50] A Cochrane systematic review (17 trials, N = 7442)[49] found that low-cost self-management programs led to small improvements in participants' self-efficacy to manage their disease, which is the principal target of the programs, as well as improvements in self-rated health status (eg, pain, fatigue, disability) and some health behaviors (eg, exercise, cognitive symptom management). However, no randomized controlled trials (RCTs) have investigated the efficacy of self-management interventions for SSc. Two before-after intervention studies of SSc self-management programs have been conducted.[51,52] One described a mail-delivered self-management program provided to 49 patients with SSc,[51] and the other was a pilot study of an Internet-delivered self-management program with 16 patients with SSc.[52] However, the small sample sizes in these studies limit the ability to draw conclusions about effectiveness. In addition, the Scleroderma Patient-centered Intervention Network (SPIN) is developing an online self-management program.[2,3] However, there are currently no SSc-specific programs readily available to patients. An alternative is a general disease self-management program, such as the Chronic Disease Self-management Program from Stanford University, which is available via the Internet. The Chronic Disease Self-management Program, which is designed to teach self-care techniques useful to persons with many chronic diseases, improved self-efficacy for disease management and overall health status in an RCT that included patients with heart and lung disease, as well as diabetes.[53]

Support Groups

A large number of patients with chronic medical illnesses, including those with SSc, join support groups in order to better cope with and manage their illnesses.[54] Activities of support groups include giving and receiving emotional and practical support, as well as providing education and information to patients. The specific activities and focus, as well as facilitator training and competence, may vary across support groups, which are typically organized locally. Patients may differ in the acceptability of the idea of attending a support group and the degree to which they may benefit from one. Because of their grassroots nature, support groups can be configured in a variety of ways.[55] For example, some support groups may meet face to face, whereas others may meet online; some groups may be facilitated by a peer, whereas others may be facilitated by a professional; and some may include structured educational activities, whereas others may not. Research on the effectiveness of support groups is scant, particularly with regard to lay-led groups. However, many people who attend support groups describe feeling more empowered, more hopeful, and less alone following their group experience.[54] In addition, some patients who attend these groups report feeling more in control of their life, as well as more knowledgeable about their illnesses, coping strategies, and developments in medical and self-help treatments.

Peer-led support groups have become increasingly popular in recent years.[56] Consistent with this, most SSc support groups are peer led rather than professionally led. However, no studies have examined the effectiveness of these groups on psychosocial or other coping-related outcomes. Given that they may be the sole source of SSc-specific support available to many patients and that they have been effective in other conditions, attending support groups may be beneficial for some patients with SSc. It is important to keep in mind that support groups are meant to complement rather than supplement standard medical care. Medical professionals may want to discuss the possible benefits of attending a support group with their patients, as well as potential pitfalls. For patients who are interested in attending or joining an SSc support group, information can typically be found on local or national organization Web sites, such as the Scleroderma Society of Canada and the Scleroderma Foundation in the United States.[57,58]

FUTURE CONSIDERATIONS AND SUMMARY

Attention and research regarding the psychological aspects of living with SSc have increased in recent years.[1,4] Furthermore, because the low prevalence of SSc sometimes precludes high-quality research in this area, the substantial progress that has been made in establishing international research networks is promising and provides a solid foundation for future research endeavors.[2,3] Future research should focus on gaining a better understanding of the psychosocial aspects of SSc, their interconnectedness, and the valid measurement of outcomes related to this, as well as on moving forward the development and testing of interventions that help patients with SSc to cope with the everyday challenges related to living with their disease.

REFERENCES

1. Thombs BD, van Lankveld W, Bassel M, et al. Psychological health and well-being in systemic sclerosis: state of the science and consensus research agenda. Arthritis Care Res 2010;62:1181–9.
2. Thombs BD, Jewett LR, Assassi S, et al. New directions for patient-centered care in scleroderma: the Scleroderma Patient-centered Intervention Network. Clin Exp Rheumatol 2012;30:23–9.
3. Kwakkenbos L, Jewett LR, Baron M, et al. The Scleroderma Patient-centered Intervention Network (SPIN) cohort: protocol for a cohort multiple randomised controlled trial (cmRCT) design to support trials of psychosocial and rehabilitation interventions in a rare disease context. BMJ Open 2013;3:e003563.
4. Malcarne VL, Fox RS, Mills SD, et al. Psychosocial aspects of systemic sclerosis. Curr Opin Rheumatol 2013;25:707–13.
5. Jewett LR, Razykov I, Hudson M, et al, Canadian Scleroderma Research Group. Prevalence of current, 12-month and lifetime major depressive disorder among patients with systemic sclerosis. Rheumatology 2014;53:1719.
6. Baubet T, Ranque B, Taieb O, et al. Mood and anxiety disorders in systemic sclerosis patients. Presse Med 2011;40:e111–9.
7. Thombs BD, Jewett LR, Kwakkenbos L, et al, the Canadian Scleroderma Research Group. Major depression diagnoses are often transient among patients with systemic sclerosis: baseline and 1-month follow-up. Arthritis Care Res (Hoboken) 2015;67:411–6.
8. Newton EG, Thombs BD, Groleau D. The experience of emotional distress among women with scleroderma. Qual Health Res 2012;22:1195–206.
9. Thombs BD, Hudson M, Taillefer SS, et al. Prevalence and clinical correlates of symptoms of depression in patients with systemic sclerosis. Arthritis Rheum 2008;59:504–9.
10. Bodukam V, Hays RD, Maranian P, et al. Association of gastrointestinal involvement and depressive symptoms in patients with systemic sclerosis. Rheumatology 2011;50:330–4.
11. Milette K, Hudson M, Baron M, et al, Canadian Scleroderma Research Group. Comparison of the PHQ-9 and CES-D depression scales in systemic sclerosis: internal consistency reliability, convergent validity and clinical correlates. Rheumatology 2010;49:789–96.
12. Van Lankveld WG, Vonk MC, Teunissen HA, et al. Appearance self-esteem in systemic sclerosis – subjective experience of skin deformity and its relationship with physician-assessed skin involvement, disease status and psychological variables. Rheumatology 2007;46:972–6.
13. Kwakkenbos L, van Lankveld WG, Vonk MC, et al. Disease-related and psychosocial factors associated with depressive symptoms in patients with systemic sclerosis, including fear of progression and appearance self-esteem. J Psychosom Res 2012;72:199–204.
14. Thombs BD, Hudson M, Bassel M, et al, Canadian Scleroderma Research Group. Sociodemographic, disease, and symptom correlates of fatigue in systemic

sclerosis: evidence from a sample of 659 Canadian Scleroderma Research Group Registry patients. Arthritis Rheum 2009;61:966–73.

15. Bassel M, Hudson M, Taillefer SS, et al. Frequency and impact of symptoms experienced by patients with systemic sclerosis: results from a Canadian National Survey. Rheumatology 2011;50:762–7.

16. Sandqvist G, Scheja A, Hesselstrand R. Pain, fatigue and hand function closely correlated to work ability and employment status in systemic sclerosis. Rheumatology 2010;49:1739–46.

17. Sandusky SB, McGuire L, Smith MT, et al. Fatigue: an overlooked determinant of physical function in scleroderma. Rheumatology 2009;48:165–9.

18. Thombs BD, Bassel M, McGuire L, et al. A systematic comparison of fatigue levels in systemic sclerosis with general population, cancer and rheumatic disease samples. Rheumatology 2008;47:1559–63.

19. Assassi S, Leyva AL, Mayes MD, et al. Predictors of fatigue severity in early systemic sclerosis: a prospective longitudinal study of the GENISOS cohort. PLoS One 2011;6:e26061.

20. Prado GF, Allen RP, Trevisani VM, et al. Sleep disruption in systemic sclerosis (scleroderma) patients: Clinical and polysomnographic findings. Sleep Med 2002;3:341–5.

21. Frech T, Hays RD, Maranian P, et al. Prevalence and correlates of sleep disturbance in systemic sclerosis – results from the UCLA scleroderma quality of life study. Rheumatology 2011;50:1280–7.

22. Milette K, Hudson M, Korner A, et al, Canadian Scleroderma Research Group. Sleep disturbances in systemic sclerosis: evidence for the role of gastrointestinal symptoms, pain, and pruritus. Rheumatology 2013;52:1715–20.

23. Schieir O, Thombs BD, Hudson M, et al. Prevalence, severity, and clinical correlates of pain in patients with systemic sclerosis. Arthritis Care Res 2010;62:409–17.

24. El-Baalbaki G, Lober J, Hudson M, et al. Measuring pain in systemic sclerosis: comparison of the short-form McGill Pain Questionnaire versus a single-item measure of pain. J Rheumatol 2011;38:2581–7.

25. Hudson M, Steele R, Lu Y, et al, Canadian Scleroderma Research Group. Work disability in systemic sclerosis. J Rheumatol 2009;36:2481–6.

26. Suarez-Almazor ME, Kallen MA, Roundtree AK, et al. Disease and symptom burden in systemic sclerosis: a patient perspective. J Rheumatol 2007;34:1718–26.

27. Benrud-Larson LM, Haythornthwaite JA, Heinberg LJ, et al. The impact of pain and symptoms of depression in scleroderma. Pain 2002;95:267–75.

28. Merz EL, Malcarne VL, Assassi S, et al. Biopsychosocial typologies of pain in a cohort of patients with systemic sclerosis. Arthritis Care Res 2014;66:567–74.

29. Frech TM, Baron M. Understanding itch in systemic sclerosis in order to improve quality of life. Clin Exp Rheumatol 2013;31:S81–8.

30. El-Baalbaki G, Razykov I, Hudson M, et al. Association of pruritus with quality of life and disability in systemic sclerosis. Arthritis Care Res 2010;62:1489–95.

31. Razykov I, Levis B, Hudson M, et al. Prevalence and clinical correlates of pruritus in patients with systemic sclerosis: an updated analysis of 959 patients. Rheumatology 2013;52:2056–61.

32. Malcarne VL, Hansdottir I, Greenbergs HL, et al. Appearance self-esteem in systemic sclerosis. Cog Ther Res 1999;23:197–208.

33. Benrud-Larson LM, Heinberg LJ, Boling C, et al. Body image dissatisfaction among women with scleroderma: extent and relationship to psychosocial function. Health Psychol 2003;22:130–9.

34. Amin K, Clarke A, Sivakumar B, et al. The psychological impact of facial changes in scleroderma. Psychol Health Med 2011;16:304–12.

35. Richards H, Herrick A, Griffin K, et al. Psychological adjustment to systemic sclerosis: exploring the association of disease factors, functional ability, body-related attitudes and fear of negative evaluation. Psychol Health Med 2004;9:29–39.

36. Jewett LR, Hudson M, Malcarne VL, et al. Sociodemographic and disease correlates of body image distress among patients with systemic sclerosis. PLoS One 2012;7:e33281.

37. Ennis H, Herrick AL, Cassidy C, et al. A pilot study of body image dissatisfaction and the psychological impact of systemic sclerosis-related telangiectases. Clin Exp Rheumatol 2013;31:S12–7.

38. Knafo R, Thombs BD, Jewett L, et al. (Not) talking about sex: a systematic comparison of sexual impairment in women with systemic sclerosis and other chronic disease samples. Rheumatology 2009;48:1300–3.

39. Schouffoer AA, van der Marel J, Ter Kuile MM, et al. Impaired sexual function in women with systemic sclerosis: a cross-sectional study. Arthritis Rheum 2009;61: 1601–8.

40. Impens AJ, Rothman J, Schiopu E. Sexual activity and functioning in female scleroderma patients. Clin Exp Rheumatol 2009;27:38–43.

41. Levis B, Hudson M, Knafo R, et al. Rates and correlates of sexual activity and impairment among women with systemic sclerosis. Arthritis Care Res 2012;64:340–50.

42. Levis B, Burri A, Hudson M, et al. Sexual activity and impairment in women with systemic sclerosis compared to women from a general population sample. PLoS One 2012;7:e52129.

43. Maddali Bongi S, Del Rosso A, Mikhaylova S, et al. Sexual function in Italian women with systemic sclerosis is affected by disease-related and psychological concerns. J Rheumatol 2013;40:1697–705.

44. Walker UA, Tyndall A, Ruszat R. Erectile dysfunction in systemic sclerosis. Ann Rheum Dis 2009;68:1083–5.

45. Foocharoen C, Tyndall A, Hachulla E, et al. Erectile dysfunction is frequent in systemic sclerosis and associated with severe disease: a study of the EULAR Scleroderma Trial and Research group. Arthritis Res Ther 2012;14:R37.

46. Keck AD, Foocharoen C, Rosato E, et al. Nailfold capillary abnormalities in erectile dysfunction of systemic sclerosis: a EUSTAR group analysis. Rheumatology 2014;53:639–43.

47. Rosato E, Barbano B, Gigante A, et al. Erectile dysfunction, endothelium dysfunction, and microvascular damage in patients with systemic sclerosis. J Sex Med 2013;10:1380–8.

48. Iversen MD, Hammond A, Betteridge N. Self-management of rheumatic diseases: state of the art and future perspectives. Ann Rheum Dis 2010;69:955–63.

49. Foster G, Taylor SJ, Eldridge SE, et al. Self-management education programmes by lay leaders for people with chronic conditions. Cochrane Database Syst Rev 2007;(4):CD005108.

50. Barlow J, Wright C, Sheasby J, et al. Self-management approaches for people with chronic conditions: a review. Patient Educ Couns 2002;48:177–87.

51. Poole JL, Skipper B, Mendelson C. Evaluation of a mail-delivered, print-format, self-management program for persons with systemic sclerosis. Clin Rheumatol 2013;32:1393–8.

52. Poole JL, Mendelson C, Skipper B, et al. Taking charge of systemic sclerosis: a pilot study to assess the effectiveness of an internet self-management program. Arthritis Care Res 2014;66:778–82.

53. Lorig KR, Ritter PL, Laurent DD, et al. Internet-based chronic disease self-management: a randomized trial. Med Care 2006;44:964–71.

54. Davison KP, Pennebaker JW, Dickerson SS. Who talks? The social psychology of illness support groups. Am Psychol 2000;55:205–17.

55. Uccelli MM, Mohr LM, Battaglia MA, et al. Peer support groups in multiple sclerosis: current effectiveness and future directions. Mult Scler 2006;10:80–4.

56. Ussher J, Kirsten L, Butow P, et al. What do cancer support groups provide which other supportive relationships do not? The experience of peer support groups for people with cancer. Soc Sci Med 2006;62:2565–76.

57. Available at: http://www.scleroderma.ca/Support/Find-A-Support-Group.php. Accessed December 10, 2014.

58. Available at: http://www.scleroderma.org/site/PageServer?pagename=patients_supportgroups#.VCeEoSi6plcss. Accessed December 10, 2014.

Index

Note: Page numbers of article titles are in **boldface** type.

Rheum Dis Clin N Am 41 (2015) 529–543
http://dx.doi.org/10.1016/S0889-857X(15)00046-0
0889-857X/15/$ – see front matter © 2015 Elsevier Inc. All rights reserved.

Printed and bound by CPI Group (UK) Ltd, Croydon, CR0 4YY

03/10/2024

01040488-0001

.